PRIVATE

AN OWNER'S GUIDE TO THE MALE ANATOMY

PARTS

Yosh Taguchi
Jan '97

YOSH TAGUCHI, M.D.

EDITED BY MERRILY WEISBORD

M&S

1st edition published in hardcover 1988
Reprinted in trade paperback 1989
2nd edition published in trade paperback 1996

Canadian Cataloguing in Publication Data
Taguchi, Yosh.
  Private parts: an owner's guide to the male anatomy

2nd ed.
Includes index.
ISBN 0-7710-9067-6

1. Generative organs, Male – Diseases. 2. Generative organs, Male.
I. Weisbord, Merrily.   II. Title.

RC 881.T34 1996   616.6'5   C95-932943-9

The publishers acknowledge the support of the Canada Council and
the Ontario Arts Council for their publishing program.

Illustrations by David D. Rolling

Typesetting by M&S, Toronto
Printed and bound in Canada using acid-free paper

McClelland & Stewart Inc.
The Canadian Publishers
481 University Avenue
Toronto, Ontario
M5G 2E9

1 2 3 4 5   00 99 98 97 96

Contents

Preface

The English edition of *Private Parts* has reached best-seller status in Canada and has been or is being translated into five other languages: French, Spanish, Japanese, Chinese, and Russian. I have been delighted not only with the public response, but with the warm reception from students and physicians. Perhaps the most flattering remark was made to me by a urologist from Western Canada. I was at a national meeting of urologists in Halifax, Nova Scotia, when a stranger approached me.

"I want to shake your hand and thank you," he said.

"What for?" I asked.

"You have done us a great service with your book. You have put our specialty on the map."

I was too stunned to get his name.

Later, the chief of medicine at my hospital asked me to make a presentation at medical grand rounds. It was a singular honour for someone in a surgical specialty. He introduced me as someone who had fulfilled every doctor's fantasy – to write a best-seller.

Seven years have passed since the first edition of *Private Parts* was published, and it is time for an update. I am proud to say there is no statement in the first edition I need to retract. (Actually, that is not quite true, there may be one statement. I suggested the seminal vesicle is a storage bin for sperm. That is not entirely correct. The fluid from the seminal vesicle does contain sperm, but it is not teeming with sperm.) But a few people have pointed out errors.

"I found a mistake in your book," my patient said.

"That's quite possible. Where is it?" I asked.

"On page ninety-four you say 'A blind man came to see me.' . . . A blind man cannot see you."

I agreed and promised to correct that in the next edition.

Another man brought me a clipping from a British paper. It was a story about the discovery of the world's largest earthworm. It measured several metres in length. This was in reaction to my statement that when I carve out the prostate I remove little pieces the "size of earthworms."

One patient called to say he had a problem not discussed in the book.

"What is it?" I asked.

"I'm too big," he replied.

Oh sure, I thought, just like the man who had called a talk show during the book's promotion to say he had a problem with his ejaculate.

"What's the problem?" I had asked, falling into his trap.

"When I ejaculate I fill a jug," he said.

"You, sir, have a vivid imagination," I remember replying.

The man on the phone now might be another joker with an ego problem. But I chose not to dismiss him.

"I cannot help you without a better understanding of the problem. You can come to my office with a Polaroid of your problem organ, or, if you prefer, you can come to the clinic and our technician can induce an erection with a drug injection."

"I will come to your clinic," the man said.

After injecting the drug, my technician called me in alarm. "You gotta see this!" he said.

The man's erect penis was 31 cm (12.5 inches) in circumference. The patient had not been playing a trick on me, he did indeed have a problem. I confessed I had never seen such a condition. The patient, a fifty-five-year-old businessman, filled me in on the details. He had had a normal sex life until his wife died some years previously. He had then been sexually abstinent for years until he met a new companion, a woman his age. He could not say exactly when his penis had achieved its present size when erect, but he was certain the problem had developed gradually. Flaccid, the penis was normal.

"We laugh about it, but, in truth, it's not a laughing matter," he said.

The erect penis was grotesquely swollen in the middle. The base of the penis and the head were normal, but the shaft was ballooned out so that his organ took on the shape of a football. I thought there might have been a blowout on one wall, with the outer skin disguising the defect, but there were no weak areas in the wall containing the erectile tissue.

I suggested we pare down the penis on its sides, leaving intact both the nerve above and the urethra below. Nerve damage was unlikely, I said, but potency could not be guaranteed. He agreed to the operation, which was relatively easy to carry out, and the results were quite acceptable to all concerned.

"Hey, I have a line you could use in your book," another patient said. "There is a vas deferens between a vasectomy and no vasectomy." It was a good line, but here is my favourite story about a vasectomy.

A patient said he was shaving his scrotum in preparation for the procedure. He had forgotten to lock the bathroom door and was confronted by his five-year-old son.

"Hey, Dad, what are you doing?" the boy asked.

"Oh, I'm just getting ready to have an operation so we won't have any more babies," my patient replied, forced to tell the truth under the circumstances.

His son, perplexed, looked at him for an uncomfortably long time. Then he said: "But, Dad, it's not you, it's Mom who has the babies!"

This edition contains new and exciting information about the prostate gland. I will discuss how management of benign enlargement is shifting from surgical to medical. I will discuss the significance of the PSA blood test for prostate cancer, and when a trans-rectal ultrasound examination of the prostate should be done. I will update the information on drugs to treat prostate infections.

I am appalled at recent suggestions that the PSA blood test has rendered the rectal examination obsolete. The blood test is better, certainly, than a hasty rectal examination that pays no heed to an asymmetry of the gland or a hard nodule. But not all cancers are going to have an elevated PSA.

A patient referred to me with "prostate trouble" had a nodule, confirmed to be a cancer on needle biopsy. His wife wanted to know why the disease had not been picked up by the company doctor he had visited before seeing his general practitioner. I suggested she visit the doctor and tell him what had transpired. She returned to tell me the following story.

She explained to the company doctor that I had done a rectal examination and known right away there was a cancer because of a hard area in the prostate.

"But all prostates get harder as men get older," the doctor had replied. (That is not so.)

"The specialist stuck a needle in and proved there was a cancer," she said.

"Ahh, they're sticking too many needles into people today," said the doctor.

Information on sexually transmitted diseases, including AIDS, is updated in this edition. And newer drugs to create an erection will be discussed.

I have also added three new chapters. A chapter on urinary tract infection compiles and synthesizes information scattered throughout the first edition; a chapter on incontinence addresses the most socially crippling problem of our aging population; and, finally, there is a chapter that discusses disorders of the kidney.

Acknowledgements

My friend Merrily Weisbord coaxed and coached me into writing the first edition of *Private Parts*, and in the process made me a better writer – so much so, in fact, that I did not need to rely on her so much this time around, a testimony to her skills. I want to thank my publisher, Doug Gibson, for permitting me to produce this second edition, and Alex Schultz, my editor at McClelland & Stewart, who assumed the role admirably executed by Patrick Crean in the first edition. Whenever I fudged or strayed, Alex set me straight, making what I had thought was clear, crisper and clearer still.

In my acknowledgements for the first edition, I thanked the people who had encouraged me to write, such as Mike Rosenbloom, J.J. Brown, and Jack Kelley. I should also have thanked Louis Dudek, who, at one time, was my English teacher.

I deliberately chose not to mention my teachers and colleagues in medicine, fearing they might not wish to have their names associated with my "private" project. The warm reception accorded *Private Parts* has changed my mind. I wish now to acknowledge Kenneth J. MacKinnon, former chairman of Urology, McGill University, who encouraged me to pursue a career in Urology, and John B. Dossetor, who got me involved in medical research. I had the added privilege of training under Andrew W. Bruce, whose distinguished career included the chair of Urology at Queen's University, McGill University, and the University of Toronto. I am proud to be associated today with Mostafa M. Elhilali, the current McGill chairman of Urology. His quick grasp of every new innovation in Urology along with his enormous managerial skills have been wonders to behold.

I would also like to name my colleagues in practice, Doug Ackman, Sam Aronson, Armen Aprikian, Michel Bazinet, Alex Brezinski, Gerry Brock, Michel Carmel, Jacques Corcos, Norm Halpern, Anne-Marie Houle, Brahm Hyams, Steve Jacobson, Irwin Kuzmarov, Mike Laplante, Doug Morehouse, John Oliver, and Simon Tanguay, as well as former colleagues who have moved on to other things, including John Foote, Magdy Hassouna, Yves Homsy, George Kiruluta, Dale McClure, Duke McIsaac, Bal Mount, Jacques Susset, John Trachtenburg, and Howard Winfield. I treasure their friendship and know that sharing discussions with them has enriched my outlook. I wish I could also name all the residents who have passed through the McGill program during my tenure, as they have all remained friends.

Finally, I want to thank my wife, Joan, and my grown-up children, Kathleen, Edwin, Jocelyn, and Carolin, for their continued love, support, and ever-reliable counsel.

Introduction

A generation ago, medical information was secret information, privy only to members of the medical profession. And the members of the guild guarded their precious secrets with a proprietary interest. The secret they didn't want out was how little they knew.

The subterfuges employed were ingenious.

"There's no point trying to explain it, you wouldn't understand. You just concentrate on getting well and leave the worrying to me."

Or:

"It's a thing-a-ma-jig."

"What?"

"What you have is a thing-a-ma-jig."

"I don't understand."

(You're not supposed to.)

The keep-'em-guessing principle was applied even to neophytes in the profession. When I was a junior intern in the Orthopedic service, I wondered why we were bandaging a wound that had already healed. I asked the chief: "Why are we applying wet sulfa dressings to a clean skin wound?"

His answer: "How often are you doing it, son?"

"Once a day, sir."

"Well, from this day forward, you will do it twice a day." (End of conversation.)

Today, there is a plethora of "How to . . . ," "Why . . . ," and "Confessions of a . . ." type books on most medical subjects, but until the first edition of *Private Parts*, a popular book on the health problems of men's private parts did not exist.

The groin area has, for years, been taboo. This was brought home to me a few years ago when I instructed young medical students to pull the sheet down to the patient's mid-thigh level before they begin a physical examination of the abdomen. By so doing, I suggested, the doctor shows the patient that he does not consider any part of the body embarrassing or sacrosanct. Furthermore, there are more health problems in the groin and genital area than there are a foot above or a foot below, and pulling down the sheet insures that this area will be examined and not passed over. Prescient advice, I thought. But I heard through the grapevine that I was out of line, that I was not respecting the privacy of citizens. Citizens yes, patients no, is my reply.

I see problems of the private parts every day, as I have for the past thirty years. As a young man, when I qualified as a surgical specialist in Urology, I was challenged by the intricacies of technique and I devised a new surgical procedure for cleaning blood in patients with non-functioning kidneys. Soon after, my interests broadened to include basic medical research, and I obtained a Ph.D. in Experimental Medicine, presenting my contributions on transplant rejection at international symposia. All this time I practised as a urologist, and because I practise under the government medicare system in Canada, I see a great many patients, many more than my U.S. counterparts. It became obvious that Urology was more than simply surgery or medicine. People came to me for help with a uniquely wide variety of sensitive and often disturbing problems. I began to take note of this and apply myself not only to medicine and surgery, but to the other very real needs of my patients for information, encouragement, and advice.

Most people, no matter how successful or intelligent, are surprisingly ignorant when it comes to bodily functions and disorders. I suspect the average man turns a blind eye to health matters – until a problem arises, and then he panics. I remember one patient, a world-renowned professor, suggesting that his abuse of chocolates was the cause of his newly discovered cancer. Another patient, a lawyer, asked me where his kidney might be. He had no idea whether the organ was in his chest, abdomen, or pelvis. A university professor asked me whether the carving-out of his prostate gland would change the sound of his voice. A businessman wondered whether he could catch his wife's cervical cancer. I have seen men turn green and faint with just a gentle touch of their genitalia. "Anywhere else, Doc, but I just can't stand to be touched there." Educated, intelligent people become inconsistent and irrational when they have to deal with health problems of their private parts.

This book is the answer to all the questions I have ever been asked – timidly, angrily, curiously – in the sanctity of my office. Questions about why urination has become painful or difficult, whether a vasectomy cuts potency, the pros and cons of circumcision. Questions about which partner is infertile, what treatments are available, and what exactly is artificial insemination. Taking care of these concerns is what I do every day. No question is irrelevant. I have been around long enough to know that private parts, although taboo, are of vital interest.

In this book I will talk as if I were talking to a friend or a patient in my office. I will explain puberty, erection, orgasm, and the workings of the prostate in such a way that you can understand how your body functions. I will discuss the old and the new sexually transmitted diseases so that you can distinguish between media rumour and real risk. I will describe surgical procedures from the point of view of a surgeon and tell you how to choose a good doctor. Many of these questions and topics affect the vast majority of men at some time in their lives, yet are grossly misunderstood. I believe that understanding what's going on in your own body will help you. From what I have seen, knowing what can go wrong and what can be done about it makes things easier.

I pull no punches. This is a straightforward, honest effort. My goal is to eliminate the traditional secrecy and make useful information easily available. If I can assuage the fears and help men deal realistically with the health of their private parts, I will have succeeded.

1

Private Parts:
What They Are and How They Work

This book is about the male body; more precisely, about that part of the male body that is covered by an athletic support. Many men refer to this part of the body as their "privates." On the outside are the penis and the scrotum, and inside the body are the bladder, prostate, testicles, and other genital structures. Often, men don't know very much about their privates – even, say, where their prostate is located. To compound the problem, they are often too timid to ask questions. Reading this book will make you more informed and relaxed about this part of your body. It will give you a sense of what's normal and what's not, what disorders can arise, and what can be done about them.

This chapter begins with a simple description of where the various parts are located in the body, how they look, and how they function in a normal, healthy man. This basic business will orient you so that you can understand the sections about your specific concerns that will be covered later on in the book.

The Penis

This organ must be the focus of more male attention than all the *femmes fatales* in the world. I see countless patients who come to my office because they are preoccupied with the size and shape of their penis. "Shouldn't it be bigger?" "Do the bags hang right?" "I was hit by a baseball when I was ten years old. Everything turned black and blue, that's why it's so small." I examine each one of these patients forthwith, and invariably I see a perfectly normal organ.

If the preoccupation with penis size did not cause such real distress, it would be funny. As it does, suffice it to say that the size of the penis has nothing to do with virility. Many men think women derive more pleasure from a larger penis, but, while it may be true that for most women the ideal man would be well-endowed, penis size is a male preoccupation. I have never heard a woman complain about the size of her partner's penis. Rigidity, or the strength of the erection, is more important to women than size. And even men with a partial amputation of the penis, due to cancer, still have pleasurable intercourse.

As a ballpark figure, the average length of the flaccid penis is 7.5 to 15 cm (3 to 6 inches), although some are shorter and some are longer. The length of the erect penis varies from 10 to 20 cm (4 to 8 inches), with the same proviso, and the average diameter at the base is about 3.75 cm (1.5 inches). Those who wish to hang on to a preoccupation with size may desist when they consider that the human penis, in relation to body size, is a paltry thing compared to those of other animals. The boar has a penis 45 cm long (1.5 feet); the stallion 75 cm (2.5 feet); the bull 90 cm (3 feet); the elephant 1.5 m (5 feet); and the blue whale 2.4 m (8 feet).

In uncircumcised men, the head of the penis, the glans, is

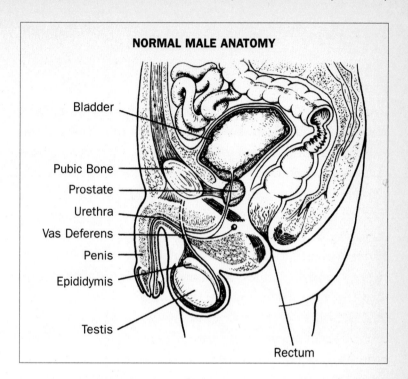

NORMAL MALE ANATOMY

Bladder

Pubic Bone

Prostate

Urethra

Vas Deferens

Penis

Epididymis

Testis

Rectum

covered by a sleeve of skin known as the foreskin. The amount of foreskin varies considerably, and there is no problem for adults as long as the foreskin can glide easily over the head of the penis. The area under the foreskin should be cleansed daily with soap and water.

The shaft of the penis is covered by smooth, hairless skin. Inside the shaft are three cylinders of erectile tissue: a pair on top, and a smaller cylinder below. This smaller cylinder contains the urethra and ends as a bulged head, which is the *glans penis*. The paired cylinders end just behind the glans and extend into the body, beyond the visible portion of the penis, to each side of the pelvic bone. The main nerve and the blood vessels run in the midline, on top, between the paired cylinders. Nerve tendrils branch out everywhere in the penis, but particularly to the head. Direct stimulation of these nerve endings produces a man's most exquisite sexual sensations.

Erection

The erectile tissue is in the three cylinders that make up the shaft of the penis. When the penis is limp, the erectile tissue is like a compressed dry sponge, with very little blood passing through. The blood that does flow into the penile artery is shunted directly into the outflow vein, by-passing the erectile tissue. When erection occurs, tiny trapdoors (named polsters) close off the shunt, and the erectile tissue fills with blood. This causes the penis to straighten out, like a garden hose when the tap is turned on and the nozzle is closed.

The polsters are activated in two ways. Sometimes sexy thoughts send a message to the polsters through the sympathetic nerves. At other times, touching, rubbing, or other direct stimulation activates the polsters through the spinal column, like a knee jerk. Morning erections are often reflex erections, activated by the stimulation of a full bladder. If they occur when the bladder is not full, obviously other factors are at play. But whatever the cause, the presence of a morning erection means that, physiologically, all systems are go.

Of course, polsters are not actual physical structures. Doctors have searched for tiny muscles in autopsy studies and come up with a blank. They are useful, however, as an explanatory concept. It is likely that chemical receptors are the polsters' physiological equivalent, as it is possible to create an erection by injecting chemicals directly into the erectile tissue.

In young adult men, the erect penis assumes an angle of 140 to 160 degrees, give or take a few degrees. This angle corresponds to the angle of the vagina. When the strength of erection is normal but the angle is less than 90 degrees, it is possible to shorten the upper surface of the penis by surgically removing wedges from the coverings of the erectile cylinders. This is done so that intercourse can be comfortable.

Intercourse

Although intercourse is not the only form of sex play between consenting adults, it is often the ultimate act. The thrusting motions massage the penile nerve endings in a rhythmic manner to create an intense preorgasmic sensation that is almost always pleasurable.

Pain is uncommon and usually due to an injury of the tag of skin that runs from the foreskin to the undersurface of the head of the penis. If this tag tears and heals with a scar, erection and intercourse can pull on it and cause pain. A simple surgical repair, or a circumcision, cures the problem. Pain that is not due to this tag of skin, or to a disease in the penis, is rare.

Orgasm

When stimulation reaches a certain intensity it triggers the waves of contractions we associate with orgasm: the bladder neck contracts; the muscles around the prostate gland, seminal vesicles, and vas deferens contract, squeezing semen into the urethral passage; the ejaculate forms a glob stretching the wall of the urethra and the muscles of the pelvis contract. The result is the pleasurable sensation of orgasm and ejaculation.

Ejaculation

It is not uncommon for normal men to ejaculate two to five minutes after penetration. Hours of thrusting and intricate sword play are more the stuff of novels than of daily life.

A man could be said to have premature ejaculation if he ejaculates before he penetrates his partner, or if he ejaculates moments after penetration. Men who experience this problem frequently consult sexologists, who have a number of techniques to delay ejaculation. Some therapy involves mental training, and some involves physical reconditioning. In one popular technique, the head of the penis is pinched by either partner when ejaculation is imminent. This aborts the ejaculation. Stimulation is then resumed. This technique is practised until a more satisfactory pattern of ejaculation is established. I have counselled a number of patients on this technique and many patients are helped by it. A similar ancient Chinese remedy consists of pressing on the perineum, midway between the scrotum and the anus, instead of squeezing the tip of the penis, to abort the ejaculation reflex. This method does work but is less effective.

Ejaculation is almost always pleasurable, causing activity in the "pleasure centre" of the brain. Painful ejaculation, however, is not an uncommon complaint. A number of middle-aged men complain that ejaculation sometimes hurts. I pay more attention to those who tell me it hurts all the time. In these cases I check for cancer or infection of the prostate gland. If the rectal examination of the prostate and the prostatic secretion are normal, I reassure the patient and suggest a heaping teaspoon of baking soda, four times a day, in a glass of water. Normal ejaculate is alkaline, and I hope that by alkalinizing the body with baking soda, the symptoms will be alleviated. Although patients' reports are positive, I am not certain whether I am treating the symptom or the psyche.

The normal ejaculate varies in volume from 0.5 mL to 8 mL (0.1 to 1.6 tsp), give or take a millilitre, and the bulk of the fluid is from prostate secretions. Sperm makes up only 5 per cent of the total volume. This explains why men who have had a vasectomy don't see or feel any difference in their ejaculate.

Ejaculate fluid is milky, sticky, highly alkaline, and has a pungent odour. This odour is not due to the sperm, as the ejaculate from a vasectomized man smells the same.

A bloody or rust-coloured ejaculate frightens most men. It may signify prostate cancer or infection, but most often it is as innocent as a nosebleed. Traditionally, men with a rusty ejaculate were treated with antibiotics, but recent studies have demonstrated that patients who don't take antibiotics do as well as those who do. I massage the prostate, produce a secretion, and treat patients only when the prostatic smear suggests a prostate infection or if the rectal examination suggests cancer.

The Urethra, Prostate, and Bladder

The Urethra

The urethra is a delicate, thin-walled tube, about 20 cm (8 inches) long. It extends from its opening at the tip of the penis to the bladder. In the penis it is enveloped in spongy erectile tissue. Near the bladder it is surrounded by the sphincter muscle that keeps urine in the bladder. Just beyond the sphincter it is surrounded by the prostate gland, and this is the site of possible prostate problems. Should the prostate enlarge, it is here that the urethra will be choked.

The urethral walls are made of unicellular "columnar" cells, which lie one beside the other, like soldiers at attention. It is only at the head of the penis that the urethral lining changes to multilayered cells like those in the skin. Because the lining is so thin, catheters and instruments can easily poke through, causing scarring and blockage in the passage. This is why doctors think twice about medical intervention. This is also why it is so astounding to discover the assorted doodads men insert into their urethras.

Over the years I have recovered a cornucopia of items from the urethra and the bladder. At different times I have extracted a safety pin, a baby onion, a glass stirring rod, and a small stick, all deliberately inserted. The items have been inserted in an ill-conceived attempt to provide rigidity or, more often, in an attempt to enhance sexual pleasure. Since objects as soft and pliable as a thin rubber catheter can irritate and damage the urethra, it's definitely best not to insert objects of any kind into this delicate passage. (I have also removed glass beads that had been surgically implanted under the skin of the penis to enhance sexual pleasure. It is not an uncommon practice in Asia, the patient assured me.)

The Prostate Gland

The normal prostate gland is about 3.75 cm (1.5 inches) in diameter, 2.5 cm (1 inch) in length, and weighs about 20 g (about 0.75 ounces). It is about as big as a chestnut or walnut and surrounds the urethra near the bladder's sphincter muscle.

Inside the prostate gland are glandular cells, muscle cells, and fibrous cells, intermixed with blood vessels, nerves, and surrounding fat. The glandular cells secrete fluid that is important for fertility, but the prostate has no vital function. Life can go on quite well without it.

In middle age, this gland has a tendency to grow and choke off the flow of urine through the urethra. Yet it can enlarge to as much as 200 g (about 7 ounces) without totally stopping the flow. Size alone is not a basis for treatment. The question really is: Does the man feel like urinating too often, day and night? Does he find his flow weak and uncomfortable? Does he have trouble knowing when his bladder has emptied? Discomfort can occur with a 100 g (3.5 ounce) gland or a

30 g (1 ounce) gland or, as is the case with half the men over fifty, not at all.

The Bladder

The bladder is the balloon-like structure situated low in the abdomen just behind the pubic bone. When empty and collapsed, it is, in size and shape, like an uncooked egg out of its shell. When filled with urine, it resembles a grapefruit or a cantaloupe. The bladder fills with urine transported by tubes called the ureters from the kidneys. A simple flap valve prevents the urine from flowing backward toward the kidney. As the bladder fills, its walls relax, accommodating the increased volume. At this point no sensations are sent to the brain. When the urine volume reaches near-capacity, the bladder registers a sensation of fullness. When it is convenient to urinate, a message is consciously sent from the brain, the bladder muscles contract, the sphincter muscle opens, and the bladder empties.

If we try to make a bladder with synthetic materials, we run into enormous engineering problems. What is required is a receptacle, like a plastic bag, that can hold more and more fluid without changing the tension in its wall, but which, when near capacity, changes into a container with tension in its wall, so that it can contract and evacuate its contents. It must have the features of a plastic bag when it is filling and metamorphose into a rubber balloon when full. Furthermore, the inner lining of the receptacle must not form encrustations despite the microscopic crystals present in the urine. The humble little bladder is a magnificent example of the intricacies of nature.

The Scrotum and the Testicles

The Scrotum

The scrotum is the skin bag that contains the testicles and their accessory structures. It is hairy and has a thin layer of muscle under the skin. When this muscle contracts, the scrotum shrinks and pulls the testicles closer to the body. When the muscle relaxes, the testicles drop away from the body. By regulating the distance of the testicles from the body, a matter of inches, the temperature of the testicles remains 1.5°C (4°F) cooler than normal body temperature. The cooler temperature is important for healthy sperm production. Bikini briefs pull the testicles towards the body and curtail sperm production. It is best to wear loose shorts, and cotton is better than nylon.

It is normal for the left testicle to hang lower than the right. Sometimes men consult me because they think the two sides should be symmetrical. They are relieved when I reassure them that there's nothing wrong. Sometimes I tell them they have a Chinese disorder. "What's that?" they ask, and I reply "One-hung-low," and we have a good laugh. If, in fact, the right testicle is lower than the left, it is indicative of a reversed position of body parts, with the heart on the right side, the appendix on the left. This *situs inversus* is part of a medical disorder called Kartagener's syndrome, which is associated with problems with the lungs. Fortunately it is very rare.

The Testicles

Normal testicles can be as small as an egg yolk or as big as a large plum. Large testicles do not mean greater masculinity or fertility. Nor does their size correspond to height or body weight.

Before birth, the testicles start life high in the back of the abdomen, near the level of the kidneys. They descend gradually as the foetus grows, and, by the eighth month *in utero*, are attached under the abdominal sac. In the final month before birth they drop further, into the bottom of the scrotum, pulling the bottom of the peritoneal lining down with them. The piece of peritoneal lining now in the scrotum is like an empty sausage casing closed at the bottom. In normal health, this tube of peritoneum closes off at the top as well. The potential opening is always present, however, and all men are susceptible to hernia formation, a condition in which the intestine is pushed into the tube.

Inside each testicle is a cluster of tubules separated by Leydig and Sertoli cells. The Leydig cells manufacture testosterone, the male hormone, and secrete it directly into the bloodstream. The Sertoli cells nourish the tubular cells, which become transformed into sperm. The transformation of a tubular cell into a sperm takes over seventy days – from the parent tubular cell, the spermatogonia, to the primary spermatocyte, to the secondary spermatocyte, where the chromosome numbers are halved, to the spermatids which develop tails to become the sperm. And this transformation is another scientific marvel.

The Accessories
(Epididymis, Vas Deferens, and Seminal Vesicles)

Epididymis

The epididymis is a comma-shaped structure that drapes over the back of each testicle, attached to it like a worm on a fruit. It is less than 1.25 cm (0.5 inches) in width and just over 2.5 cm (1 inch) long. It has a head on top, a body in the middle, and a tail below. When it is cut open, there is a cluster of tiny tubules inside. If the tubules are dissected out, they form a continuous tube. Within the epididymis, the sperm mature and acquire the ability to swim. Sperm recovered from the head of the epididymis cannot swim and are unlikely to create a pregnancy, while those recovered from the tail are much more fertile.

Vas Deferens

The vas is a tube continuing from each epididymis that conducts the sperm towards the seminal vesicle. It is about as thick as a wire coat hanger and over 30 cm (1 foot) long. If the vas is cut open, the inside canal is hard to find as it is so small. The vas is almost all muscle, making it a hard cord easily felt through the scrotal skin. It takes the sperm on a long ride from the tail of the epididymis, up above the pubic bone, and back behind the bladder, to join the seminal vesicle.

Seminal Vesicles

The seminal vesicles are irregular-shaped structures, each about the size of a cigarette, lying above the prostate, behind the bladder. They are connected to the vas in a Y form so that a single duct, called the ejaculatory duct, drains both the vas and the seminal vesicles into the urethra. The seminal vesicles secrete a gelatinous fluid that forms part of the ejaculate. They also produce a sugar found in fruit, called fructose, which is found nowhere else in the body. In infertility testing, if the ejaculate contains no fructose, it means that the man was born without seminal vesicles and is irrevocably infertile.

Since the groin and genital areas of the body have long been unmentioned and unmentionable in polite society, locker-room gossip and embellished anecdotes have too often been the source of information.

"Jimmy says that you can go bald playing with your pecker."

"How did he learn that?"

"Charlie told him that's how his uncle got bald."

Locker-room dialogue may be cute for teen films, but it is no help at all for learning to live with, and care for, your body. We all need real information for the changes and challenges of everyday life. This basic anatomy walk-through is only the beginning, and now we can go on to consider each of your specific concerns about every aspect of your private parts.

2

Impotence

Psychological Causes

My patient was a retired sixty-six-year-old man with the wrinkled, weathered complexion of a seasoned sailor.

"There are so many people here waiting to see you, and I'm not sick like them. I shouldn't be wasting your time. . . . It's just that my lady friend expects so much more," he began.

"You're not altogether dead down there, then," I replied, knowing that the reason for the referral was impotence.

"No, but it disappears on me so quickly, you see, before I can do anything."

"I understand."

"To be honest, I shouldn't be complaining. I've had my share in my lifetime, more than my share in my youth, I suspect. I can live with the memory. But it's kind of hard on my lady friend, you see. She does everything possible to help me, bless her. She rubs me, licks me, sucks me, anything to get it up. Her secret powder works some, but I was hoping that you doctors might have something more to offer."

"Secret powder?" I asked. "Is it something you mix in a drink?"

"No, no! You sprinkle it on. It prickles and burns a bit, but, as I said, it helps."

"I've never heard of the preparation," I confessed.

"No kidding? Would you like to see it?"

"You have it with you?"

He said not another word but dug deep into his trouser pocket and extracted a worn envelope held together by a rubber band. He removed the strapping and unfolded the envelope carefully. I felt party to a conspiracy. He might have been showing me contraband opium or hot jewellery. I was spellbound.

"May I see it?" I asked, my hand already extended.

He pushed the envelope in my direction, still silent. Triumphant.

The powder was coarse, lemon tinted, and speckled with dark green flakes. I examined it closely, then brought it to my nose. There was an odour I recognized immediately. I suppressed a smile but could hardly contain myself.

"Well, if it helps, I wouldn't knock it," I said, and passed him back the powdered chicken stock, the parsley flakes clearly evident.

I checked my patient thoroughly and ordered a series of tests. He was not on any medication associated with impotence, he had normal sensation in the genital area, and his blood hormone levels were normal. But tests showed poor circulation to the penis, indicating a physical basis for this man's impotence. Yet he had responded, somewhat, to the "secret powder," demonstrating, even in this case, the power of the psyche.

It is estimated that twenty million American men suffer from impotence, and, traditionally, most impotence – as much as 90 per cent – is considered to be of psychological origin, often attributed to the high levels of distress in our society. Many men live competitive and stressful lives. They are often driven by images of material success and sexual prowess. Unrealistic expectations are fuelled by a barrage of sexual innuendo – on billboards, in magazine ads, and on television commercials. Success is often equated with money and sexual performance. It is not surprising that the prime example of an impotent patient is the highly successful business executive driven beyond the bounds of comfortable behaviour into impotence. In fact, 90 per cent of chief executive officers of major corporations are said to suffer from impotence.

Sometimes an individual confides that he is potent with one partner but not with another. In this case, psychological factors are at play. And even if the case is not as clear-cut as amorous preference, the task is often to discern and neutralize the psychological disturbances.

Psychiatrists keep busy with suicidal, depressed, and schizophrenic patients. Urologists are busy with surgical corrections. Thus, impotence and other psycho-sexual problems, such as premature ejaculation and inability to ejaculate inside the vagina, have become the domain of sexologists.

Sexology is a relatively new discipline. The therapeutic principle discovered and promoted by Masters and Johnson is called sensate focusing. It involves the patient and his partner in a gradually progressing program beginning with non-genital touching. The couple is encouraged to focus on general rather than genital sensation, deliberately delaying activities that might promote performance anxiety. Gradually they progress to mutual masturbation, and finally to intercourse. In the undiluted Masters and Johnson treatment, both partners, regardless of the perceived problem, undergo an intensive two-week therapy with the help of both a male and a female sexologist. But in many cities this full therapy is not available. Most sexologists work alone, with weekly appointments at best. Often the patient is alone. The sexologist may use erotic literature, videotapes, and techniques of direct counselling as well. Sexologists to whom I have referred patients tell me that when the patient is strongly motivated to recover his potency, has a co-operative partner, and is willing to make a series of visits with his partner, the results are most often satisfactory. It is important to be sure that the sexologist is a specialized psychologist, trained in a centre such as the one pioneered by Masters and Johnson.

How do we know whether impotence is due to psychological or physical disturbances? There are three main categories of physical disturbance – circulation based, hormone based, and neurologically based – and it is necessary to consider these possible causes of impotence before deciding that the problem is psychological.

Impotence from Impaired Blood Flow

One of the first potential causes of physical impotence that I check for is reduced blood flow to the penis. Sometimes the small vessel that carries the main blood flow is blocked by a blood clot or by plaque from hardening of the arteries. In this case there is no gangrene as occurs in the leg, nor infarct (death of tissue from lack of blood) as occurs in the heart, lung, kidney, or brain. There is enough blood flow to keep the penis alive, but not enough to create an erection.

The man affected usually experiences total impotence, with loss of morning erection, but no loss of libido (sexual desire). Often he also has symptoms of circulatory problems in other areas of the body, such as previous heart attacks, strokes, high blood pressure, diabetes, or elevated blood cholesterol.

The test used to pin down the diagnosis of a circulation-based impotence is the Doppler flow study. In this test, ultrasound waves are bounced off red blood cells as they flow through the artery. The ultrasound detects red blood cells in the same way sonar detects objects under water. Different patterns are recorded according to the density of the red blood cells. The ultrasound pattern obtained from the penis is compared to the pattern derived from the leg or the arm. If there are significantly fewer red blood cells in the sound pattern from the penis, the patient has an impaired blood flow.

Results from the Doppler study, however, are very much operator dependant. The positioning of the probe on the penis and its angle in relation to the blood flow can affect results. Furthermore, blood flow into branch arteries may be measured rather than blood flow into the deep artery of the penis, the only important vessel. A recent refinement called the Colour Doppler can distinguish arterial flow from venous flow, but the test requires that the patient be injected with a drug that stimulates an erection.

Another way to map circulation is to inject dye directly into the artery. This is called an angiogram and is the way the circulation to the heart is tested before a coronary by-pass operation. It is also the way the blood flow to the leg is tested before a blocked artery in the leg is replaced by synthetic tubing. The dye injected into the artery is a colourless fluid that shows up like bone on an x-ray. But this angiogram kind of "mapping" of the circulation is not normally done on the penis. The problem is that the dye needle might dislodge plaque from the arterial wall and further block the blood flow. We do angiograms only on young men, therefore, and only if they have no heart disease and if their problem is an injury that might have damaged the artery to the penis. These are the candidates who can be helped by microsurgery and so we do the angiogram to pinpoint the blockage. If the angiogram finds a blocked artery it can be corrected using techniques like those used for coronary by-passes. In coronary by-pass surgery, a vein is taken from the leg. One end is sewn into a hole made in the healthy part of the artery, then the vein is extended beyond the blockage and the other end is sewn into the heart vessel. The vein, then, bridges the blockage. When the penis has to be re-vascularized, the technical challenge is much greater, as the artery is considerably smaller. A small artery that extends from the groin to the abdomen and is not essential to normal functioning is taken down from the abdomen and sewn into the penile artery, increasing the blood flow. The vessels are so small that they can be joined only by working under the microscope, which is why this procedure is called microsurgery.

Another surgical technique being explored to correct circulation-based impotence is tying off some of the veins that take the blood out of the penis so that more blood remains within it. Dr. Ronald Virag of France has pioneered this approach, and others who have tried the technique have reported varying success. The venous circulation adapts to any interruption by creating new vessels very readily, so I am not surprised that even when there are early successes the long-term results are less satisfactory.

Impotence Due to Hormone Deficiency

Hormones are chemicals released directly into the circulatory system. They affect our physical and psychological state. When the level of the male hormone testosterone is abnormally low, there is often a loss of sex drive and the onset of impotence. Although this is largely true, it cannot be assumed that the loss of libido is due to hormone deficiency, or that depressed hormone levels will always be associated with loss of libido. I have seen men with zero-level testosterone after having their testicles surgically removed to control prostate cancer yet with their libidos and potency intact. Eventually these men become impotent, but how they could be potent for weeks with zero-level testosterone is inexplicable.

The bulk of the hormone testosterone is made in the testicles, while a lesser amount is made by the adrenal gland. The testicle need not be large and firm to be a healthy hormone producer; tiny, shrivelled-up testicles, perhaps useless as sperm producers, may be quite adequate as hormone producers.

It is not clear when and why the testicles stop producing testosterone if they have not been damaged or removed. There is no equivalent of the female menopause in men. Nevertheless, when testosterone is not being produced it can simply be replaced with periodic injections. Two hundred mg of a testosterone such as Delatestryl, given intramuscularly every four weeks, assures normal male sexual potential. Testosterone in pill-form has not been popular because of potential liver damage. Recently, an oral preparation called testosterone undecanoate (Andriol) has been introduced. It is reported to be safe as far as the liver is concerned and has had lengthy trials in Europe. Forty-mg pills are prescribed three times a day. The monthly cost, however, is considerably more than the cost of the injection.

Impotence Due to Nerve Damage

Diabetes and specific nerve diseases of the genital area can produce neurological disorders that affect potency. When impotence is neurologically based it is likely to be associated with other symptoms. The bladder or the bowel may not work well. There is likely to be a loss of sensation in the genital area. The anal sphincter is likely to be lax. And the reflex called the *bulbo-cavernosus* reflex – which causes the anal sphincter to contract when the head of the penis or clitoris is squeezed – is likely to be lost.

Impotence is always only part of a systemic nerve damage. But major systemic nerve disease can exist without impotence. It is fascinating that a man who is paralyzed below the waist, or paraplegic, is not necessarily impotent. His erection, however, comes exclusively from the mind, since he can't feel sensation in the penis. And not only is he able to have an erection, he can also experience orgasm, ejaculate, and become a father. This is because the local reflex arc from the penis to the spinal cord can be intact, and chemical receptors in the blood vessels are not diseased. Impotence due to nerve damage occurs when the nerve involved in the reflex arc to the penis is damaged or destroyed. Such injuries are common with surgical procedures such as total removal of the prostate because of cancer. Why it should occur with a simple carving out of the inner prostate tissue is more difficult to explain, although electrocautery, used to control bleeding, is presumed to be the culprit.

Impotence Related to Drugs

Drugs for the treatment of high blood pressure, drugs to counteract psychiatric disorders, and drugs to counteract anxiety disorders often cause impotence. So do nicotine and alcohol. Nicotine constricts small blood vessels and alcohol depresses all sensation, including sexual sensation. Any person who can associate the beginnings of impotence with starting a new medication should discuss the problem with his doctor. It would be unwise simply to stop taking the medication, but it may be possible to substitute another drug.

If you have erection problems associated with a new medication it may be helpful to look through the drugs listed below. I have identified them by their generic names followed by their trade names in brackets.

Drugs to Treat High Blood Pressure

Five per cent of patients taking hydrochlorothiazide (Hydro-Diuril, Esidrix, Neo-Codema), ethacrynic acid (Edecrin), or furosemide (Lasix) report impotence. Just over 20 per cent of patients on spironolactone (Aldactone) report decreased desire and impotence. Impotence with methyldopa (Aldomet) is dose related – 10 to 15 per cent if the dosage is under 1 g, 20 to 25 per cent when the dosage is 1 to 1.5 g, and 50 per cent when the dosage is 2 g a day. Guanethidine (Ismelin), when taken at dosages of more than 25 mg per day, causes retarded ejaculation in 50 to 60 per cent of patients, 60 per cent report decreased desire, and 10 per cent report impotence. Hydralazine (Apresoline) at dosages of more than 200 mg per day is associated with decreased desire and impotence in 5 to 10 per cent. Propranolol (Inderal) in high doses such as 160 mg per day is associated with impotence. Clonidine (Catapres) causes decreased desire and impotence in 10 to 20 per cent of patients.

Antihypertensive treatment has been shifting from diuretics and beta-blockers to calcium channel blockers (Adalat, Cardizem) and ACE (angiotensin converting enzyme) inhibitors (Vasotec, Capoten). Unlike the diuretics and beta-blockers, these latter two types of drugs are not associated with impotence.

Drugs to Treat Psychiatric Disorders

Among the drugs used to treat psychiatric disorders, haloperidol (Haldol) causes impotence in 10 to 20 per cent; monoamine oxidase inhibitors (Marplan, Nardil, Parnate) cause impotence in 10 to 15 per cent and delay ejaculation in

25 to 30 per cent; tricyclic antidepressants such as imipramine (Tofranil) and amytriptyline (Elavil) cause impotence in 5 per cent; lithium (Lithane) is associated with impotence in a small percentage of patients.

Anti-Anxiety Pills

Anti-anxiety pills such as diazepam (Valium, Vivol) and similar drugs can increase or decrease desire and can cause impotence, especially when taken in high dosages.

Miscellaneous Drugs

A decrease in sexuality has also been reported with a number of other medications such as cimetidine (Tagamet), used for stomach ulcers; clofibrate (Atromid-S), a drug used to treat high cholesterol levels; digitalis (Lanoxin), essential for treating heart failure; antihistamines (Benadryl, Chlor-Tripolon), used for hay fever and other allergic conditions; and anti-cholinergics (Pro-Banthine), used to treat an overly active bowel or bladder.

The Practical Management of Impotence

I treat patients referred to me with impotence no differently from all my other patients. I take the history and carry out a physical examination. By the time I have finished the examination, I will have decided whether the impotence is likely to be psychological, physical, or a combination of both. I do not claim to be always right in my judgement calls, but it isn't critical, because there is room for corrections.

If I judge that the patient has impotence of a psychological origin, I send him to the sexologist. The others have blood drawn to measure testosterone and blood sugar and are sent for the Doppler flow study. Before the results come in, I prescribe

2 mg Yohimbine tablets, 8 mg (four tablets) per day, increased to 16 mg per day. Yohimbine is now available as a 5.4 mg tablet. I prescribe it three times a day for a week, with an option to repeat for up to one year. I tell the patients the pills are not hormones or placebos, that they are safe, and that they appear to help about one patient in three or four. I suggest that they stop the pills if there are any undesirable side effects and that they should not expect a response until they have reached the 16-mg-per-day dosage. I also suggest that if the Yohimbine pills do not work, the patient might consider a month trial of desyrel (Trazodone), a drug used to treat depression, and if that doesn't work either I move on to injection treatments wherein vasoactive drugs are injected directly into the penis. Almost all patients who are not helped by either pill opt for the injection treatment.

A number of drugs to create an erection (prostaglandin-E1, papaverine, phentolamine, and atropine) have now become available. In stubborn cases a combination of several of these drugs or all of them mixed in a cocktail can be used.

I choose a deliberately small test dose of prostaglandin-E1 (Prostin VR) when a neurological cause of impotence is suspected, and a larger dose when a circulatory cause is likely. The first dose of prostaglandin-E1 might be 0.1 mL or 0.4 mL. The preparation is injected directly into the mid-shaft of the penis, deep into the side wall, using a very thin tuberculin needle. The pain is minimal. Erection occurs in about ten minutes and lasts fifteen minutes to one hour. The dosage is then adjusted up or down according to the results. Once the best dose has been ascertained, the patient is instructed to prepare the injections and to administer the drugs himself. Prostaglandin-E1 is sold as a 2 mL vial containing 50 mg per mL and must be stored in a refrigerator. Papaverine is sold as a 2 mL vial, containing 65 mg of the drug, and phentolamine comes as 5 mg of powder.

The powder is reconstituted in sterile water. In Canada, papaverine costs under $2 a vial, phentolamine costs close to $20, and prostaglandin-E1 costs $60 per 4 mL vial. Thus, when cost is a problem, I use only papaverine. This is less satisfactory as prolonged erections lasting more than six hours and scarring at the site of injection occur more often with papaverine than with prostaglandin-E1.

I have used the injection treatment to treat impotence associated with diabetes, to treat psychological impotence, and to treat nerve-related impotence after removal of a cancerous bladder or prostate. Although the dose requirements are quite varied, the treatments are highly successful. I still recall the very first patient I treated with a drug injection into his penis. He was a professional man, intelligent, rational, and he could not fathom how a minute injection of a chemical could restore function to an organ that had not worked for over ten years. When the erection did occur, tears of joy welled up in his eyes and trickled down his cheeks. I was deeply moved, and I paid silent tribute to Dr. Brindley, the British doctor who started it all. The drugs used to create an erection were used long before official approval by the U.S. government's Food and Drug Administration or by the Canadian government's Health Protection Branch. Prostaglandin-E1 in powder form, a drug called alprostadil, made by the pharmaceutical firm Upjohn, has now been approved in the United States. It will not require cold storage, and as it will come dissolved in saline rather than alcohol, it will sting less. The Upjohn product will be called Caverject and come in 20 mg vials. The price has not yet been announced.

The injection treatment does not work in all patients, nor do all patients find injections acceptable. At this point, some patients will decline further treatment. Others are anxious to try a vacuum pump or penile implant.

Vacuum Pumps

The vacuum pump was invented by an engineer. It is based on an elementary law of physics that states if you remove air from a closed chamber, something will try to replace it. Thus, if a flaccid penis is loaded inside a cylinder which is made airtight against the skin, and the air within the cylinder is evacuated by a pump, blood will be drawn into the penis. When a sufficient amount of blood has been drawn into the penis and the penis is erect, the equivalent of a tourniquet is slipped off the cylinder to grasp the penis at its base to hold the blood in the organ. The vacuum is then released and the cylinder removed. It is advised not to leave the constricting ring on the penis for more than thirty minutes. Medically approved hand-operated vacuum pumps sell for about $300. Battery-operated ones sell for about $500. Sex shops sell less fancy but satisfactory vacuum pumps for about $75. One bonus of the vacuum pump is that regular use may increase the blood flow, and there are numerous instances of restored potency due to the device.

Penile Implants

An impotent man who has tried everything and is still impotent may consider a penile prosthesis. The idea of placing a rigid splint inside the body of the penis to counteract flaccidity may not seem so outrageous if you consider the whale and the dog, each born with a bone in his penis. Early attempts to splint the human penis with rib bone were not very successful, however, since the bone tended to erode through the penis and break the skin.

Penile prostheses became a practical solution with the development of silastic – a material that combined silicon and rubber. Silastic is so inert that the body does not form scar tissue around it. If other forms of foreign matter were implanted in the penis, its tight network of fibrous cells, like the tendon of a muscle, would create a rigid non-pliable lump. The first prosthesis, called the Small-Carrion prosthesis after the doctors who developed it in 1973, was a rigid rod that filled two of the three compartments that make up the erectile body of the penis. It was immensely successful from day one, but the permanently erect penis was difficult to conceal. Most patients strapped the penis to the abdomen and coped quite well.

Newer generations of prostheses have now flooded the market. I have had most experience with the Finney flexi-rod. This prosthesis has a soft spot so that the penis can hinge down under normal circumstances. At the time of sexual activity the penis is hinged up by either partner. The prosthesis provides sufficient rigidity to satisfy sexual expectations. There are prostheses that have flexible silver wires built in so they can be bent up or down, and prostheses whose girth and length I can custom make in the operating room by peeling off the outer silastic layers or cutting off an end. The prosthesis made by Mentor, which hinges up and down, is perhaps the one most used today.

There are also several models that allow the penis to be normally flaccid but capable of being pumped up. The soft, hollow chamber of the prosthesis is connected by tubes to a reservoir of water surgically placed in the lower abdomen. A pump is installed in the scrotum and, by squeezing the pump a few times, water is directed into the prosthesis, making it rigid. A release valve restores the flaccid state. The system is not foolproof: tubes can leak, cylinders can fill up unevenly, and valves can fail.

The latest versions of the prosthesis-with-pump are self-contained units. By pressing the prosthesis in one spot, fluid is

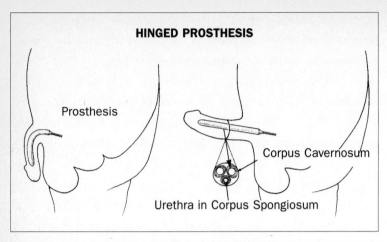

HINGED PROSTHESIS

Prosthesis

Corpus Cavernosum

Urethra in Corpus Spongiosum

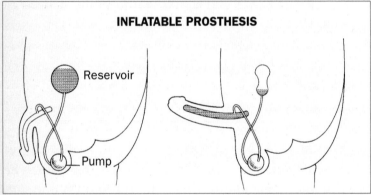

INFLATABLE PROSTHESIS

Reservoir

Pump

directed from one chamber to another, creating rigidity or flaccidity. Under the strain of sexual acrobatics, however, the apparatus has been known to collapse.

Slicker models will continue to challenge the market, but the price is skyrocketing. The self-contained pump models, for example, cost about $3,000 U.S.

I have inserted over a hundred prostheses of all varieties, and only once have I been requested to remove one. The patient became a widower and was certain he had no further use for the prosthesis.

Men who have had their potency restored by the prosthesis

experience pleasure and achieve orgasm with ejaculation. The prosthesis, in other words, is not simply an apparatus to ensure the partner's satisfaction, or to restore a bruised male ego. Some patients have fathered children. In rare instances, if a degree of potency was present before, it may augment what is provided by the prosthesis. Patients have been almost universally pleased with the results.

The Implant Operation

The penile prosthesis can be inserted in less than an hour, and the procedure is considered a relatively minor operation. In some centres, the recipient can have the operation done as an out-patient, but I prefer to admit my patients.

I have used different skin incisions (a cut at the base of the penis, a circumcision cut, or an incision behind the scrotum), but a 2.5-cm (1-inch) cut in the midline, at the point where the penis meets the scrotum, provides the easiest access. I cut the skin, then clear away the fat to expose the thick lining of the erectile tissue (*corpora cavernosa*). I incise the lining of the erectile tissue and easily insert a metal dilator into the spongy tissue. I then slip in a prosthesis of the right length and close the opening like any other incision. The only departure from routine operative procedure is the use of copious amounts of antibiotic solution to wash the inside of the erectile tissue of the penis and the incision itself to reduce the risk of infection. A catheter that is normally inserted at the beginning of the operation is left in overnight. The pain and discomfort following the operation vary considerably from patient to patient. My patients are normally hospitalized for one to three days. Pain-killing pills are usually necessary for two to eight weeks. Intercourse can be attempted at any time after two weeks but most patients are not ready for approximately eight weeks.

In the early years of this operation, while performing the procedure I could count on a number of visits from curious colleagues. I remember a visiting female anaesthetist remarking: "You never know when my husband may need one of these things!" Now the procedure has become so routine that there is no longer a flow of visitors.

Sex-Shop Items

What about sexual aids sold in sex shops or by mail-order houses?

It is fairly well established that ginseng, Spanish fly, vitamin E, zinc, and multi-vitamin preparations are of little benefit in restoring potency.

I have already mentioned vacuum pumps, but cock rings may also help certain men. A cock ring is like a tourniquet encircling the base of the penis and scrotum to retain a fleeting erection. It is slipped on after an erection has been achieved and holds the blood in the penis to keep it erect. There can be problems if the ring is left on too long; thirty minutes is considered an appropriate length of time. I advise patients who can achieve an erection but can't maintain it to wrap a rubber band around the base of the penis. If erection can be sustained, I recommend they buy a cock ring at a sex shop.

Sex After Sixty

Everybody knows that adolescent boys can get an erection and ejaculate with minimal stimulation and have another erection within minutes. After age sixty or thereabouts, a man's erection may be less firm, and he may need several days to reachieve it.

Sex after the age of sixty has been a taboo subject. When Alfred Kinsey did his pioneering research in the 1940s, he did not probe the sex life of men and women over sixty. Masters and Johnson also overlooked this population when they collected information on sexual behaviour in the 1970s. This reluctance, shyness, or modesty is somewhat endearing. But times have changed and the taboo has dissipated.

In 1992, Father Andrew Greeley reported on his survey of the sex lives of close to six thousand men and women over age sixty living in Chicago. Thirty-seven per cent of couples were having intercourse once a week, 16 per cent more than once a week. I once presented these figures at a medical conference, and the moderator, who was Turkish in origin, commented that the figures could not possibly apply to the native Turkish people, who, he said, were much more active. A woman in the audience jokingly commented that she should consider Turkey as a country in which to retire. Remarks about sexual prowess can enliven exchanges at any meeting. My statement in the first edition of this book, and repeated in this chapter, that 90 per cent of chief executive officers suffer from impotence prompted my Canadian publisher to contact one hundred CEOs across the country and ask for their reaction. The responses ranged from: ". . . is full of BS," to "the statement is libellous," to "that's quite possible," to "I'm happy to report I'm in the 10 per cent."

Is there truth in the statement, If you don't use it, you'll lose it? By and large, this is so. Men who are abstinent for a long time lose potency. Women who are sexually inactive develop contracture of the vaginal passage, lubricate less, and can find intercourse painful.

Sex is different in the older population. In the male, the erection is weaker and requires more direct physical stimulation to achieve and sustain, reaching orgasm takes longer, and reacquiring an erection takes much longer. In the female, the lack of estrogen makes the genital skin thinner and scantier. This exposes the clitoris more, reducing sensitivity or causing unpleasant tingling or prickling. Does the female lose sexual desire after menopause because the estrogen and progesterone are no longer produced by the ovaries? Not really, because the hormone that controls sexual desire in women as well as in men is testosterone.

I don't pay much attention to the age of a patient when I offer treatment, but oral preparations seldom work in the older male and I may not bother to try them. Injections are the most frequently used option, the combination of prostaglandin-E1, papaverine, and phentolamine being the standard medication. Vacuum pumps are the next most popular treatment, followed by the prosthesis.

Questions and Answers

- **What do I do if I can get an erection but it doesn't last?**

In younger men this problem is almost always psychological and a sex therapist can be very helpful. In older men this is not an uncommon problem. Some experts feel that excess venous drainage is the main problem and recommend surgically tying off some of the veins in the penis. The procedure can be successful, but not in all instances. A number of men have discovered that they can prevent a premature loss of erection by choking the base of their penis with a rubber band. In these cases a cock ring, sold at sex shops, may work.

Drug injections into the body of the penis will likely become the treatment of choice because they work.

• **How are injections into the penis done?**

The drug of choice is prostaglandin-E1 (Prostin VR). I inject 0.15 mL as the usual first test-dose. The preparation is injected directly into the mid-shaft of the penis, deep into one side wall, using the full length of the tuberculin needle. This drug stings more than papaverine but is much safer in terms of sustained erections and avoiding scarring at the site of injection. On the negative side, prostaglandin has to be kept refrigerated, and, in Canada, a 4 mL vial costs $60.

When there is no response, I try a mixture of prostaglandin, papaverine, and phentolamine. The papaverine is sold as a 2 mL vial, containing 65 mg of the drug, and phentolamine comes as 5 mg of powder. I dissolve the powdered phentolamine in 1 mL of sterile water. Four mL of prostaglandin is mixed with 2 mL of papaverine and 1 mL of phentolamine. The first test dose might be 0.3 mL of the combination. Erection usually occurs in about ten minutes and lasts half an hour to two hours. The dosage is then adjusted up or down according to the results. The patient is then instructed to prepare the injections and to administer the drugs himself. In Canada, papaverine costs under $2 a vial, phentolamine costs close to $20, and prostaglandin $60 for a 4 mL vial. Thus, when cost is a problem, I may use only the papaverine. This is less satisfactory, as the erection is not as strong and the risk of prolonged erection higher.

I have used the injection treatment to treat impotence associated with diabetes, to treat psychological impotence, and to treat nerve-related impotence after removal of a cancerous bladder or prostate. The treatments are highly successful regardless of the cause of impotence.

- **How can I travel with prostaglandin-E1 if it has to be kept refrigerated?**

Patients have told me they have travelled with the drug vial wrapped up and stored in an unbreakable Thermos bottle.

- **Isn't the injection into the penis very painful and aren't there complications?**

The shaft of the penis is not overly sensitive. A tiny needle is used and most patients are surprised at how painless the procedure can be. There is a risk of infection, but the chances are remote. Of greater concern is the risk of a scar forming within the penis at the injection sites, causing curvature on erections as described in Peyronie's disease on pages 45-7. Sustained erection, well beyond two to four hours, occurs from time to time in 1 to 5 per cent of patients. This has been called priapism, but it is different from that condition in that there is no pain. Untreated, these cases develop all the complications associated with priapism (loss of oxygenation and scarring of the spongy tissue), thus sustained erections associated with drug injections are treated like cases of priapism. First, an antagonist drug is injected. This is adrenalin as a one-in-one-thousand solution. If the erection does not go down, the compartment within the penis containing the erectile tissue is drained and washed out with a salt and heparin solution. In cases where the erection still persists, a surgical drainage procedure is carried out.

Painless prolonged erection, infection, and scarring inside the penis are possible complications, but, so far, they are very rare consequences of injection treatment. The injection treatment has been done in large numbers only for the past few years. Later complications from the repeated injections are possible, and I am beginning to see more and more cases.

I have no qualms about recommending injection treatments for impotence, however, despite these potential problems.

- **How good are pills and hormone shots for impotence?**

Yohimbine, a preparation made from the inner bark of an African tree, and originally touted as an aphrodisiac, is now being used to alleviate impotence. Yohimbine has an effect similar to phentolamine, which blocks the outflow of blood from within the blood vessels. It is, therefore, not surprising that it helps 20 to 30 per cent of patients with mild impotence. The pill is sold as a 2 mg tablet and as a 5.4 mg tablet. I prescribe the 5.4 mg tablet three times a day for one week, with an option to repeat for up to one year if it is effective.

Some people have tried testosterone preparations taken by mouth, but these preparations have to be taken in very large dosages and can injure the liver. A new drug called testosterone undecanoate (Andriol) may be less harmful to the liver, but I have had little experience with the product. Testosterone may be appropriate when the patient's blood serum shows a low level of the hormone, but in this case intramuscular injections make sense.

Impotence has also been helped by placebos; that is, pills that contain no active chemical. The healing qualities are taken on faith and faith seems to work sometimes.

- **I'm diabetic. Is impotence normal for my condition?**

Diabetes is the single most common disease associated with impotence. The exact reason is unknown. Diabetes has been related to premature aging, a sixty-year-old diabetic encountering some of the health problems normally associated with someone twelve years older. The blood vessels of diabetics are particularly subject to degenerative changes. These changes can be seen in the blood vessels of the eyes, which show changes such as those seen in arteriosclerosis. Impotence in diabetics may be circulatory in origin, although this has not been established.

I treat diabetic impotent men with the prostaglandin injections first. If there is no success, or if the patient is not happy with the response, I suggest a penile prosthesis.

- **Should I consider a penile prosthesis for my impotence? Will I be doing it for my partner or for myself?**

A man with a prosthesis has the same sensual sensations as he would with a natural erection. The operation does not disturb the nerves carrying sensation. Thus, the feeling in the penis is unaltered. Pleasurable orgasms can be expected by both partners.

- **Can a woman tell if a man has a prosthesis?**

No woman can tell from sensations in the vagina. A knowledgeable person can feel the difference with their hands.

- **How do I decide between an inflatable or a non-inflatable prosthesis?**

Basically, it is a matter of cost. The self-contained inflatable prosthesis costs about $3,000 U.S., and the non-inflatable variety costs less than $1,000 U.S. Cosmetically, the inflatable is preferable because it is less prominent under clothing, but functionally there is no difference.

- **How soon after having surgery for a penile prosthesis can I have sex?**

This depends on pain and discomfort, and these are somewhat variable. Most patients are not functional for about two months. After two weeks there is little risk of damaging either the wound or the prosthesis, but most patients are reluctant to have sex until they are completely comfortable.

- **Can the prosthesis be removed?**

Removal of the prosthesis is a very minor procedure and can be done in the doctor's office. Natural erection will not return because the erectile tissue will have been damaged.

3

The Penis

Circumcision

Should a newborn baby boy be circumcised? Parents whose religion offers them a choice will get mixed advice from the medical profession on this subject. The arguments advanced *against* the procedure might be as follows:

a. The procedure constitutes unnecessary surgery with no medical or hygienic justification.
b. The uncircumcised head retains more sexual sensitivity.
c. The foreskin may prove useful as a source for skin grafting.
d. An accident may occur during the procedure, leaving the infant mutilated.
e. The American Academy of Pediatricians (in 1971) and the American College of Obstetricians and Gynecologists (in 1978) have declared circumcision medically unnecessary.

Doctors who *favour* circumcision at birth refute these arguments as follows:

a. How can circumcision be considered unnecessary when cancer of the penis, phimosis (inability to retract the foreskin over the head), and paraphimosis (when the foreskin gets retracted beyond the head and cannot be returned) can only occur in uncircumcised men.

b. The idea that the uncircumcised head is more sensitive may be faddish and overrated. Men who have undergone circumcision in adult life do not report a noticeable difference in sexual enjoyment.

c. The number of times foreskin skin grafts have played a significant role in the health of a patient is inconsequential.

d. Mutilation of the penis during circumcision is a freak accident, like an amputation of the wrong limb. It can happen but cannot be advanced as solid argument.

e. Ask any man who has had to undergo circumcision as an adult if they would not have preferred the procedure at birth. Ask the patient with cancer of the penis. Most urologists, I suspect, favour circumcision on newborns; seeing a case or two of cancer of the penis can affect one's outlook significantly.

I have always thought it peculiar that the Academy of Pediatrics and the College of Obstetricians should make pronouncements on the merits of circumcision – they are not the ones who see problems with the foreskin in the adult male. Recently, in 1989, the American Academy of Pediatrics changed its stance. It now declares that circumcision should be a matter of choice.

One might guess that circumcision is a simple procedure since ritual circumcisions are done by mohels of the Jewish religion without formal surgical training. Newborn baby boys are often circumcised by pediatricians a few days after birth in hospital by the bell-clamp method without an anaesthetic. In the bell-clamp procedure, an apparatus that looks like a thimble is put over the head of the penis, and the foreskin is pulled over it. A second part of the instrument then clamps down on the foreskin against the thimble and cuts the foreskin off. Every baby cries lustily throughout the ordeal but I am not certain whether the infant is objecting to the strapping or the clamp.

When I was in training, I remember a senior urologist telling me that in a pinch any doctor can perform a circumcision. As specialists in the field, he suggested, we should be prepared to offer more. The procedure he recommended removes skin but nothing more. If an analogy is made to a down-filled jacket, we can shorten the sleeve by slicing off the end, such as in the bell-clamp method, or we can cut the outer material and the lining and push the filling up in the sleeve. By leaving behind the tissue between the outer and inner skin, we leave behind the vessels and nerves. There is less discomfort, less chance of bleeding, and earlier return to normal function. One doctor on whom I carried out such a circumcision told me he was sexually functional in two weeks. It is a technique I have employed throughout my professional career.

Ornery Foreskins and Other Problems (From Priapism to Cancer)

Phimosis

Phimosis is a condition affecting uncircumcised men in which the foreskin cannot easily be pulled back to a position behind the widest part of the head of the penis. The condition is associated with excess foreskin. It can also develop after an injury has torn the skin and healing has contracted the foreskin.

The simplest and only acceptable remedy is to carry out a circumcision. It is also possible to stretch the narrow opening or to slit the foreskin vertically on top, but they are inferior methods of treatment since they risk causing recurrent problems.

If there is excess foreskin but the foreskin glides easily over the head of the penis, there is no medical need for a circumcision. The area under the foreskin should be cleaned daily with ordinary soap and water. Poor hygiene, however, is not always due to sloppy habits. There is considerable anatomical variation, and a person born with a marked excess of foreskin will have difficulty keeping the area clean, no matter how fastidious he may be.

Paraphimosis

A paraphimosis occurs when a tight foreskin is pulled back behind the head of the penis and cannot be returned. The tight ring created causes the rest of the foreskin to swell, compounding the problem. If the situation is not corrected rapidly there is progressive swelling and the enormous collection of fluid distorts all normal anatomy. The solution is to squeeze all the fluid out of the area and to gently return the foreskin to its original position. When this is not possible, the skin is slit at its point of constriction so that the foreskin can be repositioned. When the swelling has subsided, a formal circumcision is advised to prevent recurrences.

Peyronie's Disease

More than two hundred years ago, in 1743, a French doctor named François de la Peyronie described an affliction of the penis that has a dramatic manifestation. Nothing much is obvious when the penis is flaccid, but upon erection the penis curves upward (and less often downward or to the left or right) ten to thirty degrees, and sometimes ninety degrees and more. (It should be noted that a healthy penis can curve ten degrees or more without it being Peyronie's disease.) When the curvature is severe, there can be pain on erection and intercourse becomes impossible. This strange condition has become known as Peyronie's disease.

In the years that have passed since the original description, we have learned some things about this disorder but nothing about its cause. No causative virus, bacteria, or chemical imbalance has been identified. What has come to light is the apparent statistical association of the condition with moderate alcohol intake, and its association with a scarring process in the hand called Dupuytren's contracture. The tendons that allow the ring and little finger to close into a fist get pulled by scar tissue, keeping the two fingers in a closed position. The tendons become prominent and obvious in the palm. A releasing procedure can be carried out by a plastic surgeon.

Peyronie's disease is scar tissue and nothing more. It involves the cover of the spongy erectile tissue. The scar prohibits expansion of that part of the spongy tissue, and erection curves the penis around the lesion. Under the microscope nothing special has been found in the scar. As in other scars anywhere in the body, calcification can occur.

Patients who develop this malady naturally fear it might be cancerous. Peyronie's disease is not a cancer and never becomes a cancer. This reassurance can be offered with confidence. Predictions about what can happen is much less certain. The condition can improve spontaneously, stay the same, or worsen.

Over the years, a number of different treatment regimens have been recommended. These include vitamin E by mouth, a pill called POTABA, injections of cortisone directly into the hard area, and X-ray treatment. One study found that leaving the patient alone was as effective as any of these treatments. I offer vitamin E to my patients (200 mg three times a day), because I know that this will do no harm.

As a rule, the disorder has not reached its final status if erection is painful or if the degree of curvature is changing. Corrective surgery should not be undertaken until the disease has stabilized, usually a period of one year. Then, if intercourse is impossible, surgical correction is considered.

Plication (a surgical pleating) of the wall of the penis opposite the scar will straighten out the organ, although the penis will be shortened. This is called the Nesbit procedure. It is simple to carry out and the results are satisfactory. The operation devised by Dr. Charles Devine and Dr. Charles Horton is also quite successful. The scar is surgically removed and replaced with a graft of the inner skin layer (called the dermis), obtained from the thigh, lower abdomen, or groin. When the condition is very advanced, as suggested by an unstoppable venous outflow of blood from the organ, the dermal graft application is not very successful. The operation may be combined with ligation of the venous outflow, but the better solution is often to insert a penile prosthesis.

Recently, promising results have been reported with direct injection into the plaque (scar tissue) of a drug called collagenase, which dissolves scar tissue. This makes sense, but more recent reports suggest minimal responses, and only in mild cases. Promising results have also been reported with injections of the drug Interferon into the plaque, but more trials are necessary before a definitive statement can be made. Laser vaporization of the scar tissue is a technique that is also being tested.

Fracture of the Penis

If the erect penis is suddenly bent, it can break just like a bone. The fracture can even emit a loud noise. Most often this accident occurs during strenuous intercourse. If the patient presents himself at the hospital, the fracture (really a tear) is immediately repaired with little consequence. If the injury is neglected, the damaged penis looks similar to that of a patient with Peyronie's disease. This has led some doctors to propose that Peyronie's disease may be due to mild injury to the erect penis that has resulted in a healing scar.

Priapism

A state of sustained, unrelenting erection, usually associated with pain and unaccompanied by any sexual desire, describes a medical condition called priapism. It must have been a doctor with some schooling in Greek mythology who first named the condition after the Greek god of fertility, Priapus. Priapus had a huge phallus, and in this sense the label is appropriate. It seems inappropriate, however, to name the condition after a god of fertility, because the end result of priapism is usually impotence and infertility.

Priapism occurs most often for no apparent reason in the sexually active male, implying, perhaps incorrectly, that extraordinary sexual acrobatics may somehow play a part. The condition can also occur when the natural flow of blood in the penis is altered by injury, drugs, or a blood disease such as sickle-cell anaemia or leukaemia. When there is a known factor promoting the condition, the disease is called secondary priapism.

The critical problem in priapism is the venous drainage system. The blood wells up in the penis, cannot escape, loses its oxygen, and promotes clot formation, then scarring.

The diagnosis is often delayed because the patient is embarrassed and fails to seek medical attention right away. Sometimes intercourse is attempted and found too painful, at which point medical advice is sought. As with most medical problems, the shorter the interval between the onset of symptoms and treatment, the better the results.

The first few hours are usually spent administering painkilling drugs, ice-water enemas, and drugs to lower blood pressure. As a rule, if there were any doubts about the diagnosis they are quickly dissipated by the failure of the patient to respond. More aggressive measures are then instituted. The hard body of the penis is pierced with a large needle. If dark, almost black blood is recovered, the penile compartment is washed out with an anticoagulant saline solution until the return flow is pink. Proper venous drainage is then established by one of several techniques. The simplest procedure is called a Winter's shunt after the urologist who introduced the technique. A biopsy needle is passed from the healthy head of the penis into penile compartment affected by the malady. This may provide an outflow channel for the trapped blood. Another technique involves re-routing an abdominal-wall vein to provide the outflow. Despite these valiant efforts, the risk of eventual impotence is substantial. So much so, in fact, that doctors treating this condition insist on covering themselves with explicit consent.

Cancer of the Penis

Men who have been circumcised at birth never develop cancer of the penis. Boys who are circumcised in their youth rarely develop the cancer. Cancer of the penis occurs virtually exclusively in men who have never been circumcised. In all probability the most vulnerable men are those who have not been circumcised and who have phimosis. Still, it is an uncommon cancer. Of all incidences of cancer in men, 1 per cent are cancer of the penis. The cancer appears as a hard lump in the penis that eventually ulcerates and oozes.

It is suspected that a peculiar bacteria called the *Smegma bacillus* promotes cancer formation. One Japanese investigator patiently and painstakingly painted the *Smegma bacillus* on rabbit penises for years but failed to produce cancer. If it had worked he would have pinned down the cause-and-effect relationship, although the fact that he didn't does not preclude the possibility. It only means that the *Smegma bacillus* may not produce penile cancer in rabbits.

When the cancer is discovered early, anti-cancer drugs incorporated into a cream such as 5-fluoro-uracil cream might control the disease. Radiotherapy can also cure the disease in its early stages. When the cancer becomes invasive, or digs in its roots, it is necessary to amputate a portion of the penis.

The portion back to one inch beyond the visible margin of the cancer is removed. Usually there is sufficient length left to allow a cosmetically acceptable result. The patient can still direct his urine stream and can resume his sex life, although it is less satisfactory when the head, the most sensitive part, has been removed. The amputated penis can look much like an uncircumcised penis, and by internal feel alone women cannot guess the length of a penis, nor whether a man is circumcised or not. The muscle of the vagina is like a rubber band that adjusts to the stretch. Men worry about the size of their penises, but, as I have said, I have never heard a woman complain about the size of her partner's penis.

Sometimes none of the penis can be retained because of the extent of the cancer. Under these circumstances the urine flow is diverted to exit behind the scrotum. Patients have to sit to urinate, but they still have voluntary control.

When the cancer is confined to the penis, the results of

surgery are quite successful. But too often the patient visits the doctor when the disease has already spread into the lymph nodes. When this has happened, a wider excision, with removal of lymph nodes, is sometimes carried out, but the results are mostly disappointing. Our hopes lie with better chemotherapy. The drugs on the market are not very effective for cancer of the penis. The highly toxic anti-cancer drug called bleomycin (Blenoxane) has been used but with limited success.

I am always baffled that a patient can come to me with the disease so advanced. More than once I have seen a man of means, immaculately groomed, accompanied by a loving wife, pull back his uncircumcised foreskin and reveal an advanced cancer with its foul dead tissue. Imagine a rotting cauliflower, that is what it is like. And the groin is filled with enormous matted nodes. How could it have been ignored to this degree?

Cancer of the Urethra

Cancer that originates in the urethra is very rare – fortunately so, because the cancer is deadly. I have never seen a patient survive it.

I recall one patient who was in his early fifties. He had difficulty passing urine, and on examination a lump could be felt inside the mid-shaft of his penis. I was a resident doctor at the time and, like the other residents, thought he had shoved some foreign object into his urethra. We were all ashamed when the lump was found to be a cancer, and heavy with guilt when he died a few months later.

Misplaced Opening

The urethra should end at the tip of the penis. Sometimes, in an otherwise well-formed penis, the urinary opening is on the shaft of the penis on top, a rare condition called epispadias.

More commonly, the opening is on the undersurface and is called a hypospadias. When the opening is almost at the head, the anomaly need not be corrected as it does not interfere with urination or reproduction. When the opening is in the shaft portion of the penis, or where the penis joins the scrotum, it is often associated with a downward curvature of the penis. This makes normal urination difficult, and intercourse impossible. A number of techniques have been devised to correct the disorder and, on the whole, the surgical results are satisfactory, both cosmetically and functionally. Success is most assured when the procedures are done on children by urologic surgeons who confine their practice to children.

Medical problems associated with the penis can be bizarre. By and large, however, the problems are routine, occasionally made more difficult by men's inhibition, embarrassment, and reticence to talk about malfunctions of their sexual organs.

Questions and Answers

- **Would you have your son circumcised?**

Yes. One simple procedure at birth circumvents a lifetime of possible problems. Apart from the fact that only uncircumcised men get cancer of the head of the penis, uncircumcised newborn boys have four times as many health problems associated with the head of the penis as do circumcised boys. In 1985, an association of urinary-tract infection with the uncircumcised state was established. It was found that uncircumcised boys were twenty times more likely to have been hospitalized for a urinary-tract infection than boys who had been circumcised. The two specialty groups that had taken a stand against routine circumcision, the pediatricians and the gynecologists, are not the ones who do circumcisions on boys or adults. Nor do they treat men with inflammation of the head of the penis, with phimosis and paraphimosis, or men dying of penile cancer. The pediatricians have changed their position: they now feel circumcision should be a matter of choice.

- **Does cancer of the penis occur in circumcised men?**

A cancer of the pigment-producing skin cells called melanoma can start in the skin of the penis. However, cancers that start at the head of the penis never occur in men circumcised at birth.

- **Does anybody ever survive advanced cancer of the penis or urethra?**

Yes, when the lymph nodes are not involved. Even cases necessitating almost total amputation, after which patients have to sit to urinate, are cured when there is no lymphatic involvement. But in my practice I have never seen a patient survive when he sought treatment only after the lymph nodes were already involved.

- **Do women get anything like cancer of the penis?**

Cancer of the vulva is the female equivalent. Both cancer of the penis and cancer of the vulva originate in skin cells. Cancer of the vulva is more common than penile cancer.

- **When I'm erect, my penis curves up and I feel a hard lump. Do I have cancer?**

If you have a history of curvature on erection, and if the lump is in the middle of the curvature, you have Peyronie's disease. Cancer never appears this way.

- **My penis curves on erection, and I'm worried about injury to my partner.**

I have heard men with very severe curvature tell me that their partners feel no discomfort. I have also seen men with minimal curvature tell me that their partners complain of pain. I doubt that it is the curvature that is the cause of painful intercourse for the partner.

- **If my penis curves to the right or to the left or downward, can it still be Peyronie's disease?**

Yes, the plaque can occur on the sides or on the underside. It occurs most often on the top, however.

- **When do I have to worry that my erection is lasting too long?**

A sustained erection is not abnormal unless the erection is painful and devoid of any desire. If it is painful, unwanted, and has exceeded four hours in duration, it is a condition called priapism. External examination of the penis cannot distinguish between sustained erection and priapism. Priapism requires prompt medical attention.

- **Why does impotence commonly occur after priapism?**

Scar tissue inside the penis destroys the ability of the spongy erectile tissue to expand. When erectile tissue cannot expand, erection cannot occur.

- **Can impotence because of priapism be treated?**

The impotence can be treated by insertion of a penile prosthesis. No other forms of treatment will work.

4

The Prostate Gland

Almost every man will get prostate trouble sometime in his life. Most often, the trouble occurs after age fifty, when more than 50 per cent of the male population develops a gradual enlargement of the prostate gland that slowly chokes off the urine flow. The cause of benign prostate enlargement is unknown, and until recently there were no pills to shrink the gland. Since eunuchs never develop prostate enlargement, there is, it seems, a causative link between testosterone and prostate enlargement. The disease is rare in Japanese men living in Japan, becomes more frequent in Japanese living in Hawaii, and is as common in Japanese Americans as it is in the white population. Thus, the traditional Japanese diet – low in fat and red meat and high in fibre – probably curtails prostate enlargement, although no tests have been undertaken to prove this. Recently, soybean products like tofu have been proposed as a protective food product. Health-food stores promote pumpkin seeds and other "natural" products as cures, but if such simple products were an effective remedy, the pharmaceutical industry would have synthesized the active ingredient long ago. In addition to pumpkin seeds, other natural products that are claimed as cures include a cactus derivative, stinging nettle, dwarf palm, African plum, aspen, purple cone-flower, and rye. An extract from the berry of saw palmetto (a palm tree found in Florida, Georgia, and Texas) has recently been touted as effective in shrinking enlarged prostate glands, but I have very little personal experience with the product. Certainly, the advertising claim that saw palmetto is every bit as good as finasteride (Proscar) and is without any side effects defies common sense.

Although not as many men over fifty develop prostate cancer as develop prostate enlargement, it has become the most common cancer in humanity and the second most-common fatal cancer after lung cancer. The cause of prostate cancer is also unknown, but genetic factors play a role. In fact, when the disease occurs in three successive generations of men, or in a father and two sons, or in brothers under the age of fifty, a dominant gene on a particular chromosome can be implicated. For some reason Afro-Americans are at increased risk for this disease.

In men under fifty, the gland commonly becomes infected with micro-organisms from the bloodstream or from the urine. Unlike infections in most other organs, prostate infection is exceedingly difficult to eradicate.

Thus, gram for gram, more health problems occur in the prostate gland than anywhere else in the male body. Given these realities, it makes sense that an appreciation and under-standing of this gland and how to care for it should rate as a high priority for every adult male.

Benign Enlargement

Symptoms

The prostate gland is situated around the urethra, and when it enlarges it begins to choke the urine flow. This creates a combination of different symptoms:

1. a slow start
2. weak flow
3. interrupted flow
4. the need to go often
5. the need to go in a hurry
6. the need to get up often at night
7. a feeling that the bladder has not emptied
8. dribbling at the end.

The symptoms develop so insidiously that older men accept the disability as part of the aging process. A slow start, particularly in the morning, is usually the very first symptom. By itself, this is not a cause for alarm. There are many men who can never void in a public washroom or on command. They need privacy, and there is nothing wrong with that.

A weak flow is one of the symptoms of prostate trouble. Often the stream is slow and stops and starts on its own accord. Slow streams and an interrupted flow mean there is a blockage. This may be acceptable to one person and unacceptable to another, so that one man may choose to have treatment and another, after getting it checked out by his doctor, may simply live with the discomfort.

Dribbling at the end of the flow is perhaps the most annoying symptom of an enlarged prostate. The flow trickles to a dribble which goes on endlessly. Imagine the annoyance of

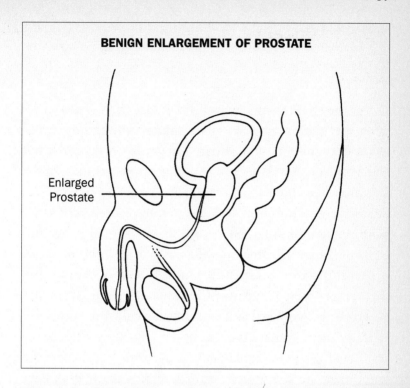

BENIGN ENLARGEMENT OF PROSTATE

Enlarged
Prostate

leaving the toilet only to find more drops coming through to wet the underwear.

The need to go often during the day and night is easily explained: the bladder is not being emptied completely at urination. This can be documented by an X-ray or ultrasound test. The enlarged prostate can also cause irritation of the sensitive neck area of the bladder. This can trigger a desire to empty. Finally, the poor flow and lack of complete emptying promotes urinary infection that can stimulate frequent urination.

If the symptoms are ignored, the story can evolve in one of two directions. There can be progressive pressure-damage to the urinary tract, eventually causing kidney damage. This is most uncommon. The more likely story is acute and total inability to pass urine. This may be precipitated by a drinking binge, a car trip when the call of nature could not be readily accommodated, or some kind of illness or surgery. There is little to match the agony of urinary retention, and its relief by catheter insertion is tremendous, as anyone who has been through the experience will testify.

Let me correct one pervasive misconception. There is no direct correlation between gland size, as detected by digital rectal examination, and urinary symptoms. A doctor is not doing his patient a favour by expressing alarm at the size of the prostate when there are no complaints about urine flow. The size of the gland is never an indication to proceed with treatment. Intervention for the benign disease should be considered only when the symptoms become sufficiently bothersome.

Recently the American Urological Association has approved a system to quantify the symptoms. Seven symptoms are scored between 0 and 5 to derive a total score between 0 and 35. Three symptoms are considered irritative: frequency of urination, urgency, and nocturia, the need to go during the night. Four are considered obstructive: hesitancy, weak flow, interrupted flow, and feeling of incomplete emptying. The more the symptom occurs, the higher the "score" between 0 and 5: 0 if it does not apply, 1 if it occurs once in five times, 2 if it occurs less than half the time, 3 if it occurs half the time, 4 if more than half the time, and 5 if almost always. When the total score is 7 or less, the symptoms are considered mild and best managed by watchful waiting; scores from 8 to 19 are considered moderate and require medical treatment; and scores over 20 are likely to require surgical treatment.

This attempt to quantify symptoms is commendable, but the figures may look more scientific than they really are. For one thing, patients tell me their scores may reflect their mood at the time. And the symptoms that are disturbing for one patient are merely annoying for another. The numbers, in other words, are not necessarily a substitute for wise judgement.

What to Do

The solution to bothersome prostate enlargement used to be surgery. If the patient was well, with no other medical problems of consequence, he just had his plumbing fixed. The routine care varied depending on the doctor, the hospital, and the region.

This has changed after startling developments. First, it was observed that benign enlargement was not as relentlessly progressive as long believed. In carefully controlled studies, as many as 30 per cent of patients reported improved symptoms after receiving placebo treatment, and other studies reported improvement with no treatment at all. Secondly, medications, called alpha-blockers, that relax the muscle cells within the prostate gland improved symptoms in 70 to 90 per cent of patients. Finally, Merck Pharmaceuticals has developed a pill that actually shrinks the enlarged gland.

Let me elaborate. It is quite reasonable just to continue monitoring a patient with an enlarged gland even if he is somewhat symptomatic. If he has to get up two or three times in the night but is not troubled by the routine, or the dribbling, he can carry on. I encourage these patients to stay away from coffee, spices, and alcohol as much as possible, and, above all, to stay away from decongestants. These "cold remedies" are non-prescription drugs and are readily available. The list includes Actifed, Benylin, Coricidin, Dristan, Drixtab, Novahistine, Ornade, Robidrine, Sinutab, Sudafed, as well as decongestants mixed with antihistamines, such as Chlor-Tripolon or Benadryl.

If the symptoms are too bothersome, I first ask my patients to try an alpha-blocker that relaxes the muscle cells. The most popular pill in this family is terazosin (Hytrin), and I have now been following patients who have been on Hytrin for several years. The drug is prescribed as a 1 mg pill at bedtime for one week, with instructions to increase the dosage by 1 mg weekly to a maximum of 5 mg. Patients are warned to be very careful when taking this medication, particularly with the very first dose. The drug can lower the blood pressure, and a very sensitive patient can experience lightheadedness or dizziness. Patients are cautioned to move very slowly if they have to go to the bathroom in the middle of the night. Despite these warnings, occasionally a patient has become dizzy or fainted. A remarkable number of patients, however, are delighted with their improved flow, reduced urgency, and reduced frequency day and night. The effects are immediate. Most of my patients are satisfied with the 5 mg dosage, although some require less and for some a 10 mg tablet is appropriate.

There are other pills that relax the muscle cells, such as prazosin (Minipress), which has the disadvantage of requiring a three-times-daily dosage. Other products in this family of drugs called alpha-blockers, like doxazosin mesylate (Cardura), will also compete for the market as they become available. Knowledgeable patients want to know if they need the Merck product as well. The answer, by and large, is yes.

The Merck pill to shrink the gland represents a fascinating story in medical detective work. A small population of men living in the Dominican Republic became known some years ago because they lacked an enzyme called 5-alpha reductase. These men never developed benign enlargement of the prostate gland. They were also pseudo-hermaphrodite, meaning that they had some female characteristics in their genitalia. At birth the boys often had undescended testes, a small penis, and small scrotum. They resembled girls early in life and were sometimes raised as girls, but at puberty they developed all the adult male features except that as they aged the prostate didn't enlarge.

The chemists at Merck became interested in how the absence of the enzyme affected the prostate. In most men the 5-alpha reductase enzyme converts testosterone into the more powerful male hormone dihydro-testosterone within the glandular cells of the prostate.

At Merck they created a molecule that resembles testosterone. The enzyme latches on to it and becomes unavailable to work on the testosterone inside the prostate cell.

Merck calls its drug Proscar (the generic name is finasteride), and figures it is a billion-dollar product. For good reason. Their market research in the 1980s indicated that 55 per cent of North American men were developing benign enlargement of the prostate gland. Of this 55 per cent, 3 per cent were having operations, 17 per cent were seeing doctors, and a whopping 80 per cent were simply living with their symptoms. If even a fraction of the sufferers take Proscar, the potential market is still enormous. Merck intends to price the pill reasonably (under two dollars for the one pill required each day) to target a large market.

How effective is the drug? It takes six months or more before any shrinkage is apparent, 4 per cent of men taking Proscar report diminished sex drive and even impotence, and the drug may not work on everybody. Merck initially claimed that in 30 per cent of patients the effects were dramatic, in another 40 per cent there were some effects but they were not dramatic, and the drug was ineffective in the remaining 30 per cent. But by 1993 Merck was claiming effective results in over 80 per cent and have since announced that men on Proscar who end up requiring surgery for relief of the obstruction can have a refund of all the money spent on the drug. This offer applies in the United States and in Saskatchewan. One major concern about the drug is that it may make diagnosis of prostate cancer more difficult because it lowers the cancer marker called PSA by as much as 45 per cent. On the other hand, if the PSA doesn't drop when Proscar is administered, this may signal possible malignancy and in fact aid the detection of cancer (as long as a PSA reading is obtained before starting the medication). Furthermore, Proscar may actually reduce the likelihood of cancer development, and it may even make bald men grow hair. The full story cannot yet be told.

If I had an enlarged prostate, would I take the pill? Yes, I would. But I might also consider other treatments that have come into the picture:

Balloon dilation, which compresses prostate tissue, is like a coronary angioplasty. The tiny balloon is placed in the urethral passage where it has been compressed by prostate tissue. When the balloon is inflated it pushes back the obstructing tissue. After about thirty minutes the balloon is deflated and removed. At best the results of this procedure last up to a few months.

Another procedure has been developed whereby a wire coil is inserted in the urethra to keep the prostate tissue from compressing the passage. These wall "stents," made of titanium, do not cause stone formation but instead become covered by normal urinary lining. They have revolutionized the management of scars in the passage (strictures of the urethra), but have not yet been perfected for handling the prostate.

Laser energy can be used to incise or excise prostate tissue without blood loss and will likely play a greater role in the future. At present, the lack of tissue for examination by the pathologist, and the fuzzy line between what needs to be removed and what needs to be left behind has limited its usefulness. Vaporization of obstructing prostate tissue with electric energy by rolling a ball over the gland is rapidly becoming more popular than using a laser, but the long-term effects are not yet known.

Variations on Proscar, anti-androgen drugs, and even the ancient estrogens may also find a role in treating the disorder.

Surgical treatment has not been totally eliminated. It will continue to have its place, although it may not remain as the second most-common operation in the United States (cataract operation is still number one). As a rule, patients who suffer from urinary retention, or a bladder stone, or infection are not likely to be helped by the medical regime, and I encourage these patients to opt for surgery.

When surgery is decided upon, my routine is as follows.

Pre-Op Tests

Before surgery, I like to make sure the kidneys are free of disease by ultrasound examination or by X-ray. A clear fluid containing a chemical with iodine is injected into a vein in the arm. Since arteriosclerosis does not occur in veins, there is no danger that the needle will release plaques, as it might in an artery. The injection, therefore, is safe, and the chemical is quickly eliminated by the kidney. An X-ray picture taken at intervals shows up the chemical in the same way it shows bone, outlining, in sequence, the substance of the kidney and the urine in the kidney, ureter, and bladder. A film taken after emptying the bladder shows the amount of urine left behind. This series of kidney X-rays is called the intravenous pyelogram (IVP). It is the single most-useful X-ray test of the urinary tract. It cannot be used in people who are or may be allergic to iodine. There is a one-in-ten-thousand chance of a fatal allergic reaction, and in practice not much attention is paid to this risk because it is so rare and because a test dose can be as dangerous as the full dose. The test is ordered with caution in people who are diabetic or have damaged kidney function. The ultrasound alternative is totally safe. Inaudible sound waves are bounced off different organs of the body and, like radar, are viewed on a monitor. An ultrasound expert can decipher these seemingly bewildering pictures with amazing accuracy and will present me with still photos of the action on the monitor along with a report, which I use to guide my diagnosis.

I check the anatomy near the prostate by direct inspection with an instrument called the cystoscope. This instrument is like a miniature periscope. The eyepiece is like that on a pair of binoculars, the shaft is about 46 cm (18 inches) long and as thick as a pencil. The instrument is inserted directly into the urinary passage, which has been lubricated and frozen with a local anaesthetic. The fibre-optic light source and micro-lens system allows very accurate examination. There may be some discomfort, but there should be no real pain. Of course the degree of discomfort will depend on the individual anatomy, any disorder, and the skill of the surgeon. The cystoscopic examination will clarify the degree of prostate enlargement and whether the right surgical approach is through the urinary passage. If it *is* the right approach, I will sometimes go ahead and do the actual operation there and then.

Without the cystoscopy, the patient is saved an unpleasant test, but there is a risk of a surprise finding at surgery, such as discovering a scar in the passage (stricture of the urethra) or a bladder tumour. As a rule, prostate surgery can be better planned with a separate cystoscopy done beforehand, but the test is considered mandatory only when blood has been detected in the urine.

Before the patient is admitted to hospital, he has more tests. These include:

1. chest X-ray,
2. electrocardiogram,

3. complete blood count,
4. serum chemistry.

These tests are routinely undertaken, because the patient's account of his illness and the physical examination may not have uncovered problems that would be hazardous with prostate surgery. For example: the chest X-ray may reveal tuberculosis or lung cancer; the electrocardiogram may show a silent heart attack or an irregular beat; the blood count may indicate anaemia or leukaemia. In some cases, the blood chemistry is out of line; the potassium may be low, the calcium may be high, or the blood sugar may be sky-high. When these pre-operative tests are normal, the patient is admitted to hospital the afternoon or evening before surgery.

As I practise in a university hospital, an intern or resident will visit, retake the patient's story, and redo the physical examination – listening to the chest, palpating the abdomen, perhaps performing a rectal examination. There are pros and cons associated with being in a teaching hospital. Some of my patients are annoyed that they have to submit to an examination by a young doctor-in-training. Some of these same patients are most grateful that a resident doctor is immediately available in their moment of distress. The resident staff is also a final check on the propriety of the operation proposed. I have, on occasion, changed my management of a case because of a new insight provided by my resident. Personally, if I ever needed hospital care, I would choose a teaching hospital because of the continual presence of the residents. Odds are, a doctor will be at your bedside faster in a teaching hospital than in a non-teaching hospital.

In the afternoon before surgery, an anaesthetist will also visit the patient and suggest the appropriate anaesthetic – a general or a spinal. The patient may have a preference because of a bad experience with one or the other, or the anaesthetist may indicate a preference to administer to a particular patient. Generals are preferred if a previous back operation complicates the chances of getting the needle into the spinal column, and in cases of heart disease, since, with a general, the anaesthetist feels he or she can better control the administration of different drugs. In most cases, however, the spinal anaesthetic is preferred because there are fewer lung complications, like a partial collapse, called atelectasis, or a pneumonia.

The Surgery

Let me describe exactly what is involved in prostate surgery done through the penis. After the administration of the anaesthetic, the patient's feet are placed in padded stirrups so that his legs are positioned like that of a woman getting a pelvic exam. The genitals are then washed with detergent and water. Sterile drapes cover everything except the penis. The urethra is lubricated and measured, and a surgical instrument called a resectoscope is introduced. The resectoscope is similar to the cystoscope but contains an electrically heated wire loop for cutting. The loop is switched on and off by a foot pedal and moved back and forth manually by finger control. The obstructing prostate tissue choking the urethra is carved out in little pieces the size of a kidney bean. When spurting blood vessels are encountered, a second foot pedal changes the electrical current, which will cauterize the bleeding vessel (electro-cautery). It takes about an hour to complete the procedure, and the bits of cut tissue are flushed out with water through the hollow tube of the resectoscope. But the prostate tissue often remakes itself after each bite of the resectoscope, much like shifting sand filling in a hole, so the skill required is not unlike that of a sculptor.

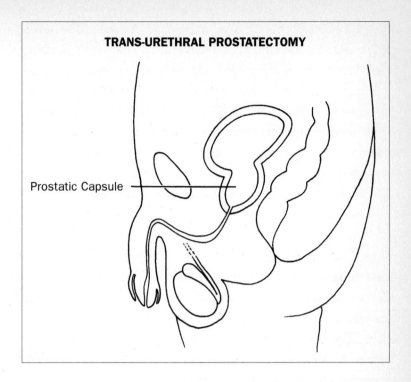

TRANS-URETHRAL PROSTATECTOMY

Prostatic Capsule

At the completion of the procedure, the inside of the prostate is a carved-out cavity. Now a soft hollow tube, called a Foley catheter, with an inflow tract and an outflow tract, is passed into the bladder. A continuous saltwater irrigation of the system is carried out for a day or two.

Prostate surgery done through the natural channel in the manner described above is called a trans-urethral prostatic resection and is the most common operation for benign enlargement. It is the least taxing and least stressful method for the patient. But it has not always been so. Trans-urethral prostatic resection was long considered one of the most difficult operations for the surgeon to learn. And it was often a bloody mess.

The development of the fibre-optic light source and

micro-lens system revolutionized this operation. Fibre-optic light allows powerful light beams to be transmitted along innumerable glass fibres made into a cord that can be twisted and bent. The micro-lens system has upgraded the optics from that of a baby Brownie to a Nikon. Forty years ago, the battery light source and the lens were such that when there was bleeding from one major vessel the procedure often had to be terminated.

As I have said, the operating time for this procedure should be under one hour, although an hour and a half is neither uncommon nor necessarily harmful. When the operation takes longer, there is an increased risk of injury to the passage (urethra) and potential formation of a scar or stricture. For the vast majority of patients, the operation takes one hour, and the catheter can come out after one or two days. After the catheter is removed, there may be considerable amounts of blood mixed with the urine for a day or two, but the flow should be better almost immediately. The patient usually leaves the hospital after four or five days.

Complications

Lung complications such as pneumonia or fluid in the lung are frequent in high-risk cases. Patients who are vulnerable include smokers, men over seventy years old, men who are more than 45 kg (100 pounds) overweight, and men with known lung diseases. Smokers have lung complications two to six times more often than non-smokers. If smokers quit three months before surgery, they better their odds.

Convalescence

During the period of convalescence that follows, most patients must accept that they will tire easily and should not overdo it. The reason for the fatigue is probably the moderate blood loss normally associated with prostate surgery. There is also a risk of more copious blood loss up to the end of about five weeks, and it's best not to travel too far away until the risk period is over.

Patients should refrain from sex, including masturbation, for two months after the operation. Ejaculation will be dry after prostate surgery, as the ejaculate is being discharged into the bladder. This is because tissue forming the neck of the bladder is removed during the procedure, which means that the bladder cannot close as it normally would, allowing ejaculate to travel backwards into the bladder. It does no harm and is eliminated mixed with urine. The sensation of orgasm is not lost.

Approximately 30 per cent of patients report varying degrees of impotence following prostate surgery, and some men are certain that the surgery is the cause. The usual explanation, however, is that the procedure is carried out on older men who normally take longer to achieve erection anyway. And men may prefer to attribute the loss of potency to a particular event in their lives rather than accepting a change in their sexual prowess. In any case most men do not suffer any loss of potency.

The patient can be home in under one week, and convalescence lasts one month. This is where the patient can play an active part in his recovery. Some doctors are very specific about the limitations imposed. For example, they may advise no stairs for two weeks, no driving for one week, no sex for six to eight weeks, and so on. I believe that the best advice I can offer is to allow the level of fatigue to guide the patient. After all, patients vary in their energy level and their ability to recuperate. Up to the point of fatigue, the more active the patient is the better. Walking is considered the best exercise, but whatever he is doing, the patient should stop and rest as soon as he gets tired. Lifting heavy objects and straining even for a bowel movement should be avoided for six weeks. High fluid intake, the equivalent of eight glasses of water a day, soothes urine flow. Alcohol, coffee, and spices are best avoided until recovery is complete, which may not be for two to three months.

It is not impossible to father a child after prostate surgery. In a minority of patients the ejaculate may shoot forward and come out the penis as usual. In the majority, the ejaculate that has discharged into the bladder can be forcefully urinated out into the vagina. More often, intercourse takes place on an empty bladder, and after orgasm the ejaculate is collected from the bladder by inserting a catheter and used for insemination. The chances of a successful pregnancy are, however, remote.

When There Are Other Health Problems

Prostate enlargement occurs after middle age, a time when there are sometimes other health considerations.

What if surgery for benign enlargement has to be considered for someone who has had a heart attack? Surgery should not take place within three months of a heart attack; the risks of a repeat attack are too high. The risks do drop off somewhat after three months, but it is wisest to wait a full six months before surgery, since the risks are then indistinguishable. It is an added insurance to arrange post-operative care in an intensive-care unit where heart function is closely monitored. With these precautions, patients who have had a heart attack can undergo prostate surgery just like anybody else. Patients who have had coronary by-pass surgery are not at increased risk, and patients who have heart-valve problems have a 20 per cent chance of heart complications.

Diabetic patients need careful management of their insulin, but diabetes doesn't mean that surgery should not be undertaken. There is, however, an increased risk of infection, because a diabetic's weak bladder muscles do not allow the bladder to empty completely.

The risk of a stroke, particularly in a patient with high blood pressure, is a concern, but even in the highest-risk group, with evidence of narrowed neck arteries, there have not been increased attacks of strokes with prostate surgery.

Other Operations for Benign Prostate Enlargement

The enlarged prostate can also be removed through an incision made in the lower abdomen. It may be decided to approach the prostate in this manner because the patient cannot be positioned for the procedure through the penis; for example, when there are severe hip problems. More often the decision is based on the size of the gland. When the prostate is very large, it may be unreasonable to expect the carving procedure through the penis to be completed within one hour.

This so-called open operation on the prostate is done in one of three ways. The oldest method is through a cut made into the bladder. This is an easy operation to perform, but is associated with distressing and painful bladder spasms. A second approach is through the opened capsule of the prostate. This is like cutting the peel of a tangerine, placing a finger under the peel and pulling out the fruit. It is often almost as easy as that, and is the procedure I favour. A third approach is to make a cut behind the scrotum in front of the anus. I never use this method as there is a risk of damaging the nerves.

These open operations on the prostate may also be selected because there is a need to carry out other corrective procedures at the same time. For example, it is possible to repair a blowout of the bladder, remove a large bladder stone, or even repair an inguinal hernia.

The stay in hospital may be a few days longer, and, as there is a cut, there is a chance of wound infection. These are minor points, and in fact there is little difference between the post-operative course associated with these procedures and the more common operation through the penis.

As far as we now know, surgery is the only definitive treatment for prostate enlargement. As frightening as surgery may be for some, prostate operations done for benign enlargement are most often quick, technically advanced, and successful. Should you need such an operation, it is wise to be mentally prepared. Awareness of what is happening to you and a positive attitude will, as in all cases of illness, aid your recovery.

Questions and Answers

- **Will I lose potency after a benign prostate operation?**

There are very few guarantees in the biological sciences. The surgery will not affect your hormone levels, the circulation to your penis, or your nerve connections. If you had no potency problem before surgery, you are unlikely to develop impotence. If you are relatively impotent, there is about a 30 per cent chance that the impotence will be worse.

- **How come I need a prostate operation when I've been told I have a small prostate?**

It is possible that you may need an operation to improve the flow, while another man with a large prostate may not. Patients have variable responses to discomfort. One man's agony is another man's distress. I suspect that some men have more elasticity in their tissue than others, and when the normal outer prostate tissue is compressed by the enlarging inner tissue, they may, therefore, have relatively less difficulty with urination.

- **Are you going to use antibiotics during surgery?**

Experts disagree on whether to use antibiotics to prevent an infection. Some feel that in the absence of a documented infection, antibiotics should not be used. Others argue that a urinary tract irritated with instruments and catheters is vulnerable to infection and that antibiotics used before and after surgery will reduce the risk of fever, chill, and dangerous kidney infections. I use antibiotics for a short period before and after surgery.

- **Will I have a blood transfusion during or after the operation?**

The amount of blood lost depends on a number of factors: the length of surgery, the skill of the surgeon, and the nature of the prostate tissue. I will have blood available and administer it when there are significant changes in the pulse and blood pressure, signalling a 20 per cent loss of the total blood volume. You should know that as much blood is lost in the days following surgery as is lost during surgery. Do not be alarmed in this period, since it takes only a little blood to colour the urine alarmingly red.

- **What are the chances that you might find an unsuspected cancer after my prostate operation?**

When there has been no suggestion of cancer on the rectal examination, there is a 10 to 15 per cent chance of an unsuspected cancer. But prostate cancer often starts in the outer part of the prostate, the part not removed in the standard carving-out process. So even when all the tissue removed shows no sign of cancer, prostate cancer can develop in subsequent years.

- **Will the prostate operation fix all my symptoms?**

In general, if the indications were correct and the operation properly done, the symptoms will improve. If the indications for the operation were incorrect, the symptoms will not be alleviated. A scar that narrows the calibre of the urethra can occur as a consequence of an injury due to the instrument or due to the catheter. This complication will produce all the symptoms of an enlarged prostate. An incomplete removal of the obstructing tissue, especially of the critical tissue close to the sphincter, will leave the patient with persistent symptoms.

- **Will I need a repeat operation?**

A repeat operation may become necessary for any of a number of reasons. For example, the first operation may have been terminated prematurely. This is an uncommon event, but even a quality surgeon will swallow his pride and stop, whether or not he is finished, when the safe time limit of sixty to ninety minutes has elapsed.

Another reason for a repeat operation might be the regrowth of obstructing prostate tissue. Men who have had their prostate operation at a young age, or who have the good fortune to live to a ripe old age, have a greater chance of requiring a second operation. About 15 per cent of patients need a second operation within fifteen years.

Unlike surgery requiring a scalpel, the repeat operation is not complicated by the first, because there is no obstructing scar tissue.

- **Does the administration of Hytrin or Proscar eliminate the need for prostate surgery or only delay the need?**

This question cannot yet be answered. It is possible that the pills may permanently eliminate the need for surgery. It is possible, also, that surgery may still become necessary. Most doctors believe that medical therapy can be tried first.

- **Will Hytrin and Proscar be necessary for life?**

I suspect most patients will start on both pills, and after some months the Hytrin will be reduced, possibly eliminated.

- **Will laser surgery eventually replace electro-cautery?**

Laser energy can vaporize the enlarged prostate tissue with virtually no blood loss. The procedure can thus be done on an out-patient basis, and can even be done under a local anaesthetic instilled into the urethral passage and by needle into an area behind the prostate.

Thus, in theory, laser prostatectomy will inevitably replace the method now used to carve out the enlarged gland. But there are drawbacks. Laser vaporization provides no tissue for the pathologist. This may be considered less important today because of the PSA test and ultrasound assessment. Nevertheless, in 15 per cent of resections unsuspected cancers are found. Furthermore, laser surgery is still less precise and less complete, although this may change with further experience. More importantly, the laser fibre costs six hundred to a thousand dollars per operation, raising questions about cost-effectiveness.

- **Will Proscar's effect on PSA limit its usefulness?**

There are some experts who feel that way, but others feel that depressed levels of PSA, no matter how they are achieved, may thwart cancer development. A PSA reading should always be obtained before starting Proscar. Normally, this reading should fall by 40 to 50 per cent in one year. If it does not, there should be a renewed search for cancer. A chemical marker released only by prostate cancer cells awaits development.

- **Is there any evidence that Proscar might reduce the risk of prostate cancer?**

The evidence is mixed and inconclusive. On one hand, Proscar has not affected the experimental prostate cancers in animal models. On the other hand, the low incidence of prostate cancer in the Japanese is associated with low levels of chemicals in the blood that reflect the degree of 5-alpha reductase activity. Men who take Proscar may develop the blood characteristics of the Japanese and may become less susceptible to cancer formation.

Cancer of the Prostate

If all men over fifty (or over forty if black or with a family history of prostate cancer) routinely had the PSA blood test along with an annual rectal examination, and if sample tissue from every suspicious prostate were taken out by an ultrasound guided needle and examined under a microscope (a biopsy), there might be a dramatic change in the death rate from prostate cancer.

It does not require much expertise to distinguish a malignant prostate from a benign one. Cancer feels hard, like a knuckle, a normal prostate or one with benign enlargement feels soft, like the fleshy part of the palm. Precautionary measures will detect 85 to 90 per cent of all early cancers. The

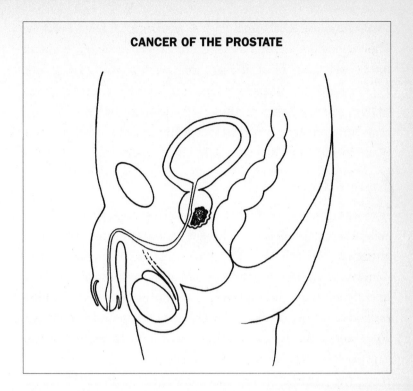

CANCER OF THE PROSTATE

other 10 to 15 per cent do not produce the firmness that can be detected by digital rectal examination or do not produce an abnormal PSA reading. In these instances early diagnosis can only be made serendipitously, if there is an associated benign enlargement sufficient to encourage prostate removal as discussed in the last section. The kidney-bean size prostate chips removed through the resectoscope and the solid masses of tissue removed with open surgery are routinely examined by a pathologist. The cancers undetected by digital rectal examination or by a PSA test are often found in this way.

The PSA blood test for detecting prostate cancer has only recently been introduced. The test involves screening healthy men for abnormal levels of prostatic specific antigens (PSA) in their blood. This is a protein secreted by every prostate cell and is responsible for making the gelatinous ejaculate liquid. The protein is secreted by prostate cancer cells at ten times the normal rate. Thus, if every man with a PSA reading over 4 nanograms/mL were subjected to an ultrasound examination of the prostate with a biopsy of sample tissue, we would diagnose early prostate cancers twice as often as by using a rectal examination alone.

Prostate Biopsy

A prostate biopsy can be done in different ways. One way is to make a surgical exposure with a cut behind the scrotum in front of the rectum. Another way is to stick a needle through the skin at a point between the scrotum and the anus with a finger in the rectum guiding the way. Yet another method, which I used to do in my office, was with a needle pressed flat against my gloved and lubricated finger, passed into the rectum to the hard spot in the prostate. The needle pierces the rectum and enters the prostate, where it collects a core of tissue the size of the lead in a pencil. The procedure takes ten seconds, and all the patient feels is a momentary jab. If the pathologist finds cancer in the specimen, no further biopsy is necessary. If the pathologist cannot find cancer, there will be concern as to whether the needle hit the appropriate spot or not.

This uncertainty about the accuracy of the biopsy has been eliminated to some extent by the ultrasound-guided needle. The ultrasound image points out the suspicious area, dots are lined up, and a biopsy gun fired. Not all cancers have the same appearance (a black or darker spot in a grey background), but the needle can be pinpointed to the selected target. When no dark areas are found, six needles into six evenly spaced areas on the outer aspect of the prostate are often done. This is called the six-quadrant biopsy.

Staging

When the pathologist sees cancerous changes in only one to three chips taken from the prostate, that is, less than 5 per cent of the tissue removed is cancerous, the disease is labelled stage A1 (or T1a). When cancer is detected in four chips or more, or more than in 5 per cent of the tissue, the disease is labelled stage A2 (or T1b).

When the cancer is diagnosed by an ultrasound-guided needle biopsy because the PSA is high, not because the gland feels suspiciously hard to the examining finger, the disease is labelled T1c, but it might just as well have been called A3.

When cancer has been detected, an attempt is then made to define the extent of the disease beyond the prostate. This will involve a bone scan, blood tests, sometimes a CT scan, and, rarely, an ultrasound examination of the liver and spleen.

The bone scan is a radio-isotope study. A chemical that emits gamma rays is injected into a vein in the forearm and finds its way into bone cells, and the radiation emitted from the chemical creates a picture of the skeleton. When cancer is present in the bone, it shows up as extra dots on the picture or as extra blanks. Arthritic joints and bones previously fractured show extra dots as well, sometimes making the interpretation difficult. A normal X-ray of the same area is often compared with the bone-scan results to clarify the problem (the radiation from the test and the X-rays is minimal). The interpretation often boils down to a judgement call aided by the results of the blood test done with it to stage the disease.

The blood is tested for markers. One marker is the PSA level. The normal level of this protein is under 4 nanograms/mL in the blood. Counts higher than this may signal the presence of cancer, although a high reading can come from an enlarged benign gland or from an infected gland (prostatitis). To complicate the picture further, as many as 15 per cent of cancer cells may not secrete this protein. Nevertheless, the PSA test is turning out to be useful in monitoring for the possible presence of cancer (screening), as well as a good test to monitor disease progression or regression, as after radical surgery, radiotherapy, or initiation of hormonal treatment.

Another well established marker is prostatic acid phosphatase, an enzyme secreted specifically by the cancerous prostate cells. Unfortunately, this enzyme cannot be detected in the blood until the disease has moved well beyond the prostate. Even when a rectal examination suggests the disease is confined to the prostate, elevated levels mean that it has spread. This enzyme can also become elevated when part of the prostate suddenly loses its blood supply, a condition called infarct of the prostate, which has nothing to do with cancer. A CT scan can see extension of the disease beyond the prostate, but not the disease spread to the lymph nodes. If stage C disease is suspected, it is likely confirmed by a CT scan.

The ultrasound test of the liver and spleen tells us whether the cancer has spread into these organs.

After involving the lymph nodes, 80 per cent of prostate cancers spread first to bones, 20 per cent spread first to the liver. Thus, in staging the disease, the doctor is guided by a battery of tests, not by one test alone. Accurate staging is the backbone of proper management. It is very important because drastically different decisions are based on the results of staging. And, again, the inconsequential amount of radiation used for these tests is not worth worrying about; it would be like worrying about the wallpaper when the house is on fire.

Stage A1 (T1a) Disease

There is considerable controversy regarding how patients with stage A1 cancer of the prostate, when less than 5 per cent of the tissue is affected, should be managed. Some centres do not distinguish A1 from A2 disease and take out the entire prostate in both cases. Other centres go back and carve out more prostate tissue before labelling the disease A1 or A2. Doctors use the PSA blood test as a guide in many other centres. If the PSA is elevated, surgery or radiotherapy is encouraged; if normal, the patient is simply monitored with regular PSA readings, perhaps every three to six months. I am guided by the PSA reading as well as by the pathologist's grading of the cancer. The pathologist commonly uses the Gleason grade, which is derived by looking for established patterns visible in the specimen at low magnification and giving the two most obvious patterns a combined grade between one and five depending on how closely they resemble established patterns. Thus, the lowest Gleason score possible is two, the highest possible is ten, and scores above six are considered serious. If the PSA reading is elevated and if the Gleason grade is over six, I treat the patient aggressively. If the PSA reading is normal and the Gleason grade under six, I simply follow the patient's progress with a rectal examination and PSA test every six months.

Stage A2 (T1b) and Stage B (T2) Disease – Operable Cancer

Patients with stage A2 cancer of the prostate, when more than 5 per cent of the tissue is affected, require further treatment. Without it the disease will spread and become fatal.

Cancers diagnosed after a biopsy is taken because the PSA reading is too high (grade T1c or A3), not because the gland feels suspicious to the examining finger, will be offered different treatments depending upon the size of the cancer seen on ultrasound as well as the appearance of the cancer under a microscope. The most likely advice is radical prostatectomy.

When cancer of the prostate is suspected on rectal examination, but the examining finger does not detect disease in adjacent organs, the disease is designated a stage B lesion. The B lesion category covers anything from a tiny nodule smaller than a pea to a lesion involving the entire prostate, sometimes further categorized as stage B2. The diagnosis is confirmed by biopsy.

When the cancer is confined to the prostate the objective is total eradication of the disease. Traditionally, one of three methods were favoured by doctors: radical surgery, radio-therapy, and radio-isotope implantation therapy.

I treat my patients with stage B1 and A2 disease with radical prostatectomy. In cases in which there is a medical contraindication to surgery, I offer them radiotherapy. I am not convinced that radio-isotope implantation with open surgery is sufficiently superior to external beam therapy to justify the rigours of the surgery involved.

Radical Surgery

Total surgical removal of the prostate is a major undertaking. The operation may take three to four hours, and there are risks of serious complications. Besides the normal risks of every major operation – the chance of pneumonia, wound infection, blood clots in the legs that may migrate to the lungs – there are risks peculiar to this procedure. There is a small risk of permanently losing urine control, but I have not yet had a patient who is totally incontinent after surgery, although many have mild stress incontinence. Most centres that do this operation frequently have total incontinence rates of about 1 per cent. The risk of permanent impotence from radical surgery used to be 99 per cent, but with the recently introduced nerve-sparing operation developed by Dr. Patrick Walsh of Johns Hopkins University, the chances of recovering potency are now 50 to 80 per cent.

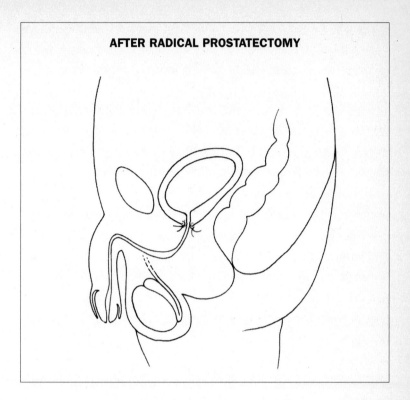

AFTER RADICAL PROSTATECTOMY

The operation starts with removal of the pelvic lymph nodes, since, when prostate cancer spreads, it always spreads here first. To date we have no foolproof way of telling if the lymph nodes are involved without first actually doing the surgery. The naked eye cannot tell if the lymph node harbours cancer or not. (A CT scan can detect lymph nodes that are larger than 2 cm [.8 inches], but smaller nodes can be cancerous.) Surgery is done and the excised lymph nodes are sent to the pathologist, who quickly freezes the specimen, slices it, stains it, and examines it under the microscope.

I rely on the frozen section reading. If there is cancer in the lymph nodes, I abandon the operation, because the disease cannot be totally eliminated by surgery when the cancer is likely in other parts of the body. I proceed with the operation to remove the prostate when the pathologist reports that there is no cancer in the lymph nodes. Two times in a hundred, the report is wrong, and the occasional false negative reading has encouraged some centres to carry out a lymph node dissection as a separate procedure, often using a laparoscope technique like that used for gall bladder surgery. I have not yet converted to this style of practice, but feel it may be appropriate when the chance of lymph node involvement is high, as when the PSA reading is over 20.

Prostate removal is one of the more difficult operations, because the area is bloody, surgery takes place in the depth of the wound, and the delicate pencil-thin urethra has to be rejoined to the wide, open neck of the bladder. If potency is to be preserved, all this must be done without damaging the cobweb-like nerves that lie just behind and beside the prostate.

The operation starts with the patient lying flat on his back and anaesthetized. The skin from the nipples to the mid-thighs is scrubbed with surgical soap and painted with an antiseptic solution. Sterile drapes cover the body except for the lower abdomen. A catheter is placed into the bladder.

I make a vertical incision that extends from the belly button to the pubic bone. Then I split the muscle below the skin in the midline, stretch it open, and am into the site for the surgery.

I dissect out the pelvic lymph nodes and send them to the pathologist for frozen section examination. The pathologist's report comes back within fifteen minutes, and depending on the result, I either continue or abandon the operation. If proceeding, I free the prostate gland on both sides and clamp and tie the large vein in front of the prostate. I can now see where the urethra enters the prostate. I cut the top of the urethra, exposing the catheter inside, and make a stitch on either side of the urethra so it won't pull apart. I take the catheter out and cut completely through the urethra. The prostate is still fixed to its bed behind and to the bladder on top. I gently dissect the back wall of the prostate upwards towards the bladder, protecting the nerves necessary for potency. I then cut the prostate away from the bladder. Next I cut away the vas and the blood supply from the back of the prostate wall. The seminal vesicles are dissected so that they can be removed with the prostate. Only now can I remove the prostate. Once the prostate is out, I fit the bladder to the small urethral opening by putting stitches in the bladder opening to make it smaller and fixing it to the urethra with four stitches, using the two stitches already in the urethra. A Foley catheter is put into the bladder, tubes are placed in the wound to drain spilled urine and blood, and the wound is closed.

I have become more selective in choosing patients for the operation. When the cancer mass is microscopic, the patients are just carefully monitored. Patients with stage B disease whose cancer occupies more than half the volume of the gland are directed towards radiotherapy. Too often the surgical margins contain cancer when the cancer mass approaches half the prostate's size, and a cure is not achieved. Thus surgery is best for those patients with cancer volumes that are between 5 and 50 per cent. Despite this restriction I have done increasingly more operations, making radical prostatectomy one of my most frequent operations. Many centres now place patients on hormonal treatment for three months prior to surgery. Such treatment can down-stage the tumour, and the pathologist is less likely to see cancer cells at the margins of the specimen. It may be that the cancer is still present but less detectable. The likelihood of this "error" is lessened by a special test called cytokeratin staining. I only pretreat my patients with hormones when there is a delay in the surgical date, especially those patients with elevated PSA readings. A trial is underway in Canada to determine whether pretreatment with hormones will better their odds.

As prostate cancer is a slow-growing tumour, it is not unreasonable to wait several months from the time of diagnosis to the time of surgery. During this period some patients donate up to three pints of blood to have on hand at the time of surgery.

I recall one patient who was not mentally ready for surgery and was placed on hormones. When the patient had his operation three months later, the pathologist could find no cancer in the removed prostate gland and had to recheck the biopsy to confirm the original diagnosis. The disappearance of prostate cancer with hormone treatment may occur in 4 to 5 per cent of cases. The idea of down-staging the cancer with hormone treatment is not fanciful, but too often it does not happen. Recently, I abandoned surgery on a patient whose lymph node showed minute cancer on the frozen section. Had that patient been on hormones, the lymph nodes might have been negative and I might have proceeded with the surgery. But would that have been better for him or worse?

Radical prostatectomy is very major surgery, and, in my estimation, one of the most challenging technical procedures because of the delicate reconstruction of the urinary tract. When there is meticulous attention to detail, there are fewer complications and continence and potency are preserved. Surgery is the treatment of choice for stages B1 and A2 prostate cancer because the results are superior to radiotherapy or radio-isotope therapy.

Radiotherapy

In radiotherapy, powerful gamma rays are directed at the prostate gland from many directions. These rays kill cancer cells more than they do normal cells, but the distinction is fuzzy. Thus, when radiation hits the skin in substantial amounts, the skin turns brown and hard. When radiation irritates the lower bowel, there can be cramps, diarrhea, and pain. Radiation injury to the bladder can contract the bladder, causing frequent need for urination, and can cause the bladder lining to bleed more readily, because surface vessels become more prominent and can break more easily.

Despite these potential problems to the skin, bowel, and bladder, most patients don't suffer, and many are helped.

With radiotherapy, the cancer is contained but often not eradicated. Biopsies taken after curative courses of radiotherapy show cancer in the original site. Nevertheless, the cancer *is* largely contained, and radiotherapy to the prostate is less hazardous and toxic to the body than radiotherapy to the lungs or abdomen.

Most surgeons believe that surgery, when possible, is more curative than radiotherapy. The cancer takes longer to return after surgery, if it returns at all. But this may simply reflect the health of the patient before treatment. Patients with early B disease are more likely to get surgery than patients with advanced B disease. Also, surgery is less likely in men over seventy.

Some surgeons feel they can down-stage C disease to B disease with hormone treatment to make surgery possible. I am not convinced this occurs with any regularity and have not recommended it.

Radio-isotope Therapy

Radio-isotope treatment was pioneered at the Sloan-Kettering Cancer Center in New York City. In this operation the prostate gland is dissected free from its surrounding tissue, and instead of it being removed, radioactive gold pellets are inserted into it. This allows doctors to use powerful gamma ray radiation without risking its complications. But it does require fairly major surgery, and the cancer is contained rather than cured.

Recently, another radio-isotope treatment has been developed. Instead of radioactive gold, radioactive palladium is used. The half-life of radioactive palladium – that is, the time when one half the radioactivity is dissipated – is much shorter for palladium than it is for gold. The radiation can thus be better controlled. These "seeds" of palladium are inserted through the skin behind the scrotum and in front of the rectum. Over seventy-five centres in the United States are presently equipped to carry out this procedure. The results have yet to be determined. I believe this method may become the treatment of choice for early cancer undetectable to the examining finger.

Stage C (T3) Disease

When the examining finger detects cancer spread to the seminal vesicle, bladder, or urethra, the disease is labelled stage C. Stage C disease is also often found by a CT scan, an X-ray that shows a mass of 2 cm (.8 inch) or more.

Stage C cancer of the prostate is often mistakenly managed like a stage B. That is, on the presumption that the cancer is only in the prostate, radical surgery is done. Occasionally we see later that the disease has spread beyond the prostate and is, in fact, a C. When we know beforehand that the disease has spread beyond the prostate, most urologists manage the patient with radiotherapy or with hormonal manipulation, as if he had stage D disease.

Stage D (N+ M+) Disease

When cancer has spread into the lymph nodes or beyond, it is labelled stage D. This category is further divided into D1

(N +), when the cancer has spread only into the lymph nodes, or D2 (M +), when the cancer has spread beyond the pelvic lymph nodes, the bone scan is positive, and the level of the enzyme released by the prostatic cancer cells (prostatic acid phosphatase) is elevated. Unfortunately, many patients with cancer of the prostate are diagnosed only at this later stage. The PSA levels in these patients can be into the hundreds or thousands.

Eighty per cent of prostate cancers are hormone dependant. This means that the cancer is stimulated by a certain hormonal environment, and inhibited by another hormone environment. Dr. Charles Huggins of the University of Chicago, working with Dr. Hodges, was the first to show this in 1941.

Prostate cancer is stimulated by the male hormone, testosterone. Thus, removal of the testicles, the main source of testosterone, can cause dramatic resolution of the cancer. An almost identical effect can be achieved by the administration of the female hormone stilboestrol by mouth; or by monthly injections of a drug that acts on the master gland (the pituitary), inhibiting testosterone production. The two drugs most commonly used are goserelin acetate (Zolodex) and leuprolide acetate (Lupron).

These three methods of achieving castrate levels of testosterone are equally effective in fighting cancer. One method is not superior to another, and combining two or three do not improve results. Orchiectomy (removal of the testicles) achieves castrate level of testosterone in two hours, stilboestrol takes about two weeks, and the monthly injections about three weeks. Stilboestrol in therapeutic doses of 3 mg per day is seldom used anymore because it is associated with increased risks of cardiovascular complications. Removal of the testicles is a minor surgical undertaking, but can be psychologically devastating. In my experience, however, the psychological effect is not that harmful. Patients with cancer are anxious to get help, not preserve body image or potency. Virtually all my patients faced with D type cancer learn to accept surgical removal of the testicles. A patient occasionally wants testicular prostheses, which are soft plastic balls that resemble testicles in size and feel. But I prefer to remove the contents of the testicles leaving the cover of each testicle behind, a procedure called subcapsular orchiectomy. All the hormone-producing cells are removed and nothing else. The testicles still have sensation, although they feel much smaller.

Testosterone is also produced by the adrenal gland, and to counteract this source, an anti-androgen pill, flutamide (Euflex) or nilutamide (Anandron), has been added to the treatment regime. These medications block the male hormones from getting into the prostate cells. The combined treatment has been called maximum androgen blockade. Dr. Fernand Labrie, of Laval University, in Quebec City, was the first to promote the treatment and the possibility that it would prolong life in cancer patients. Further studies from around the world failed to confirm this claim initially, but patients and doctors alike will try anything that improves the odds, and more recently figures have indicated that maximum androgen blockade does improve survival figures, perhaps by between six months and a year.

In Canada and in Europe, a single oral medication with the potential to provide maximum androgen blockade is quite popular. This drug is cyproterone acetate (Androcur). Critics claim that cardiovascular complications – like those associated with stilboestrol (inflammation of the veins and blood clots to the lung) – as well as the eventual progression of the disease occur more often with this regime than with the anti-androgen combined with removal of the testicles or Zolodex/Lupron injections. Proponents of Androcur claim the addition of small amounts of oral stilboestrol (0.1 mg) overcomes these shortcomings. Megestrol acetate (Megace) will compete with Androcur for the market. It is less expensive but has a shorter track record.

Hormonal manipulation will not affect the 20 per cent of prostate cancers that are not hormone dependant.

All patients with stage D cancer are monitored with periodic blood tests (PSA and, sometimes, acid phosphatase), rectal examinations, and bone scans. Eighty per cent of patients will feel better, with less bone pain and weight loss. There will be a corresponding improvement in the bone scan picture and in the blood picture. Sometimes the remissions are life long.

When, despite adequate hormonal treatment, cancer progresses after a period of remission, it is designated D3 disease, and the prognosis becomes grim. Most of these patients survive less than one year, and until recently we had very little to offer them. Cortisone treatment helped some, as did radioactive strontium, but most patients were given palliative pain-control medication only.

Some promising results with new combinations of old drugs and brand new drugs are beginning to be reported. By and large, these treatment trials apply only to patients who are active and otherwise well. One approach uses estramustine phosphate (Emcyt), a pill that works like estrogen and also has an anti-cell division effect, combined with intravenous Vinblastine, an established cancer chemotherapy agent. Equally promising results are being reported for a combination of Emcyt and Etoposide, an anti-cancer drug that can be taken by mouth. These regimes cause hair loss and possible bowel and blood disturbances, but as many as half the patients respond, and a few have complete response, meaning the spread lesions in the bones disappear. Dr. Ken Pienta, of Detroit, has pioneered these treatments.

Another approach combines ketoconazole (Nizoral), an anti-fungal agent that suppresses testosterone, and weekly intravenous doxorubicin (Adriamycin), a long-established cancer chemotherapy agent Drs. Nicolas Bruchovsky and Larry Goldenberg, of the University of British Columbia, have early results suggesting that the hormone therapy on an on-and-off cycle may achieve better results, as the time off therapy keeps the cells resistant to hormones from proliferating.

Prostate cancer has become the most common cancer in men, affecting approximately 9 per cent of the male population. The incidence is rising 2 to 4 per cent annually. Although more people die of lung cancer, prostate cancer may soon overtake it to become number one. At the hospital in which I work, new cases of prostate cancer are diagnosed more often than lung cancer, breast cancer, and cancer of the cervix combined. It is true that most men survive prostate cancer, but 25 to 30 per cent do not.

Prostate cancer is curable if diagnosed early, and even with a late diagnosis, it is controllable to some extent.

Because more patients with prostate cancer die from natural causes than from an uncontrolled progression of the disease, another treatment option has been gaining support, particularly in the lay press. This option is to do nothing but wait and monitor the patient, reacting only to obvious progression of the disease or the development of pain. Dr. Willet Whitmore, former chief at Sloan-Kettering, probably initiated this debate over treatment when he wondered aloud whether treatment is necessary when prostate cancer is curable, and whether a cure is possible when treatment is necessary. This question, widely known as Whitmore's conundrum, makes the point that prostate cancers that progress are often indistinguishable from those that do not. Obviously, radical prostatectomy is unwise for a disease that may not progress, and is equally unwise if surgery does not produce cures. Recent figures are starting to show, however, that surgery for the aggressive early disease (high grade) can cure, that surgery which leaves behind cancer cells at the margins is unprofitable, and that "masterful neglect" can lead to an earlier demise. The trend towards involving patients more and more in the decision-making process cannot be faulted, but there is a limit. After all, anyone who treats himself has a fool for a doctor. Ask yourself: Are there any health problems where early diagnosis and early treatment translate into poorer outcomes?

Questions and Answers

- I know a PSA reading over 4 is above normal, but does a count over 10 mean cancer is likely?

Not at all. PSA readings over 10 can be associated with benign enlargement or prostate infection. Neither is a PSA reading of under 4 the standard for all men. It has recently been proposed that the normal count for men under fifty should be less than 2.5; less than 3.5 for men aged fifty-one to sixty; less than 4.5 for those sixty-one to seventy; and less than 6.5 for men between seventy-one and eighty.

- How is the ultrasound examination of the prostate done?

The patient is prepared with an enema the night before and started on a three-day course of antibiotics one day before the test. After undressing, the patient lies on his side on the examining table. A probe, about the size of a thumb, is inserted into the rectum. The tip of the probe is often covered with a sac filled with water over which there is a condom. When the probe is activated, it is like turning on a flashlight that produces sound waves instead of light. The prostate is seen as the sound waves bounce off it. The early cancer shows up as a dark area on a grainy grey background. A needle that is fixed to the probe can then be guided through the rectal wall into the spot. The entire procedure may take fifteen to twenty minutes.

- **Even if the cancer has spread beyond the prostate, shouldn't you remove the prostate anyway?**

The Mayo Clinic is exploring radical prostatectomy, plus removal of the testicles, in cancers that have spread into the lymph nodes but not beyond. The long-term results of this approach are still not known. If it is true that new deposits of cancer can come only from the original site, there may be some merit to this approach. Experimental studies have shown, however, that spread lesions can come from spread lesions.

I have used the Mayo approach in treating a few of my patients, but time alone will tell whether it is justified. Critics of the approach argue that equal or better results may be achieved with hormonal treatment only.

- **Do I need hormone pills after a radical prostatectomy?**

If the surgery has removed all the cancer cells, no further treatment is necessary. Every six months, follow-up tests are done. The PSA blood test and a rectal examination have replaced routine bone scans, abdominal ultrasound, and CT scans.

- **If there is recurrence of disease after radical prostatectomy, is radiotherapy preferable to hormonal therapy?**

If the recurrence is at the margin of the surgery, and if potency is prized, radiotherapy would be the first choice. If disease is seen on a bone scan, hormonal therapy would make more sense.

- **I've had an orchiectomy (removal of the testicles) and I take anti-androgen pills. The cancer seems to be under control, but can anything be done for the hot flashes?**

Taking a small dose of stilboestrol (0.1 mg) by mouth or substituting a progesterone type pill (Androcur or Megace) for the anti-androgen can eliminate the problem.

- **Is subcapsular orchiectomy as good as total orchiectomy?**

There are no hormone-producing cells (Leydig cells) in the outer part of the testicle, nor in the epididymis. Tests have shown that testosterone level achieved with subcapsular orchiectomy is the same as that obtained with complete removal of the testicles. If I had the problem, I would opt for a subcapsular orchiectomy.

- **I'm in my late seventies. Is there any point in my being checked for prostate cancer any more?**

Some experts will say that after age seventy-five or eighty, testing for cancer can cause more harm than good. Why create anxiety, they say, when it is an unlikely cause of death? This argument is valid if one can accurately predict a person's life span. If a patient has less than ten years of life ahead, it is unwise to investigate the prostate for potential cancer. If such a prediction cannot be made, it would be a mistake to deny the testing, especially if the patient seeks it.

- **I have been told I have a pre-malignant condition after a prostate biopsy. Should I get a second opinion?**

When the pathologist reads the specimen as showing prostate intraepithelial neoplasia (PIN), it is considered a pre-malignant condition. A second opinion is unnecessary, but careful follow-up is essential.

- **Can the pathologist be wrong in his diagnosis of cancer?**

This is most unlikely. When the pathologist is uncertain, he or she will say what those misgivings are and examine more sections of the specimen. When the pathologist says it's a cancer, it is, unfortunately, a cancer.

- **I have been reading more and more articles suggesting that routine PSA testing and routine rectal examinations do more harm than good. Is that true?**

The issue is philosophical. When my patients raise this question, I answer by drawing an analogy to maintaining a car. Do routine visits to the garage prolong the life of an automobile or shorten it? If the mechanic tampers and bungles, he is likely to have done more harm than good; if he detects early trouble and addresses it, the car may last longer. Similarly, if a doctor tampers with a body that should have been left alone, it may be harmful. On the other hand, if he detects early disease and offers curative treatment, life may be prolonged.

Prostate Infection

Of the three common maladies afflicting the prostate gland – namely, benign enlargement, cancer, and bacterial prostate infection (prostatitis) – prostate infection is the most frequently misdiagnosed, mistreated, and misunderstood. First of all, there is no clear understanding of why prostate infection occurs. We know that an invasion of the bowel bacteria through the bloodstream and into the prostate causes infection and inflammation of the gland. This describes the route of infection, but we don't know why prostatitis occurs in some people and not in others. There seems to be no sexual association; people who do not have sex get bacterial prostatitis as often as those who do.

Although a venereal cause is remotely possible, the micro-organisms associated with prostatitis are usually not of that variety. The vast majority of cases of prostatitis have no sexual implications. Like bacterial infections in other organs – tonsillitis, bronchitis, or meningitis, for example – micro-organisms settle in a particular part of the body because there is a specific predisposition, or sometimes, for no good reason at all. The prostate may be predisposed to infection in someone who, for whatever reason, is regularly bounced about while sitting on a hard surface. Indeed, prostatitis has long been called the "jeep driver's disease." Constipation has also been suggested as a predisposing factor. By and large, however, no specific causative factor can be found. In my practice I have found patients uniformly agreeing to one thing: "Yes, I have been working too hard and not getting much sleep. And, yes, I have been under considerable stress of late." In other words, prostatitis is a disease of our times.

Whatever the reason, bowel bacteria, most often *Escherichia coli*, settle into the prostate. The illness then takes one of two forms. Either there is an acute illness with high fever, chills, prostration, and difficulty with urine flow, known as acute prostatitis; or there is a vague malaise, itchy urethra, discomfort in the area behind the scrotum and in front of the anus (called the perineum), and perhaps some discomfort on urination, known as chronic prostatitis.

Acute Prostatitis

Acute prostatitis may require hospitalization, intravenous fluids, and powerful antibiotics, but the clinical course of the illness is relatively short, with complete and total recovery. The diagnosis is not difficult to establish; micro-organisms are almost always seen in the urine and blood. A routine culture of the urine and blood confirms the diagnosis. Traditionally, medical students are taught not to subject patients to repeated rectal examinations. On first exam, the infected prostate will be hot and tender, and pressing on it is like squeezing an infected pimple; there is a risk of pushing micro-organisms into the blood-stream.

Once in a while a patient will not respond to even the most powerful drugs, and there will be persistent high fever. An abscess of the prostate is likely. This condition is best treated by allowing the abscess to drain into the urinary passage. The instrument that is used to carve out the prostate in cases of cancer or benign enlargement (a resectoscope) is used to create the drainage.

Despite the ominous nature of some of the remarks made here (concerning powerful drugs, high fever, surgical drainage, and so on), acute prostatitis is almost certainly curable.

Chronic Prostatitis

Chronic prostatitis, on the other hand, can linger so long it has driven men to utter despair. Constant low back pain, a continual urgent need to urinate, disabling discomfort in the rectum or lower abdomen, loss of libido, and impotence are persistent symptoms that may make life seem not worth living.

But chronic prostatitis is frequently misdiagnosed. A patient may be saddled with the diagnosis with little supporting evidence. He may have some discomfort that he can feel is in the area near the prostate, he may find urination uncomfortable and frequent. These symptoms may all arise from anxiety and have nothing to do with any physical disorder.

Bona fide chronic prostatitis can also be misdiagnosed. The doctor may presume he is dealing with a psychosomatic disorder and not take the steps necessary to establish the diagnosis.

The diagnosis cannot be made from the patient's history, nor from examination of the urine. I believe that only by carrying out a vigorous prostatic massage with the gloved and lubricated finger in the rectum, to express fluid which is collected from the tip of the penis, and examining it under the microscope, can the doctor rule in or rule out the diagnosis of chronic prostatitis. If a patient has the disorder, the doctor will see more than fifteen white blood cells, often in clumps, under a microscope set at forty times magnification. Patients without the disorder will have fewer than fifteen white blood cells. Period.

The massage is distressing and often painful for the patient. (I am, as a result, unconvinced that the prostate constitutes an erogenous zone. On the other hand, there is not much doubt that the anus can be.)

I once suggested to a gathering of doctors that examining the expressed prostatic secretion under a microscope was mandatory to diagnose chronic bacterial prostatitis. A doctor in the audience asked what he should do if a microscope were not readily available. I was baffled, but the technique is not commonly accepted and is very infrequently performed. Subsequently, I began testing the expressed secretion with a leukocyte (white blood cell) strip on a dipstick. I discovered that almost all patients with chronic bacterial prostatitis have an elevated reading. The correlation with the fifteen or more white blood cell count was extraordinary and I am in the process of preparing a scientific report.

I must say, using a microscope is not the accepted way to establish the diagnosis of chronic bacterial prostatitis. Drs. Meares and Stamey proposed the academically approved test long ago. Their method was to take a bacterial count on the first drops of urine passed, another count on a specimen collected after the first 10 mL, then bacterial culture of the fluid expressed by prostatic massage, and, finally, a bacterial count on the urine sample obtained after the prostate massage. When the bacterial count in the specimen obtained after massage exceeded the first and second specimen, the diagnosis of chronic bacterial prostatitis is established. The test is obviously very elaborate, time consuming, and not always feasible. Patients often cannot void the separate specimens on demand. That is why I choose to base my diagnosis on the microscopic analysis of the expressed prostatic secretion.

Treatment consists of both general and specific measures. General measures include: high fluid intake to flush the system; hot baths to encourage more circulation to the area; and regular ejaculations, which have the same effect as periodic prostatic massages. Alcohol, coffee, and spices are restricted if not eliminated. They are all irritants causing tissue swelling, and their use is like adding gasoline to a fire.

What the doctor does specifically is prescribe antibiotics. The problem is that there is a blood-prostate barrier; that is, few antibacterials diffuse from the blood stream into the prostate. Two products that do are the trimethoprim-sulfamethoxazole combination, called Septra or Bactrim, and the antibiotic Erythromycin. Erythromycin is not very effective against bowel micro-organisms like *E. coli*, which is the most common bacterial cause of prostatitis. Its efficacy can be improved by adding baking soda to the regime. The baking soda helps to make the body fluids more alkaline, and thus creates a better environment for the drug. The trimethoprim-sulfamethoxazole combination has been the most effective and most commonly used medication. The usual dosage is a double-strength pill taken twice a day.

Second generation tetracyclines, like minocycline (Minocin) or doxycycline (Vibramycin), are considered effective by some experts. The ordinary tetracycline has to be taken on an empty stomach to be fully effective, loses potency when taken with milk, can cause teeth discoloration, and can make the patient sensitive to direct sunlight, something equivalent to snow blindness. All these problems are eliminated by the more expensive second generation of the drug. But it seldom eradicates chronic prostatitis and is therefore not the drug of choice.

The quinolone family of drugs, such as norfloxacin (Noroxin), ciprofloxacin (Cipro), and ofloxacin (Floxin), are rapidly establishing themselves as the drugs of choice for this condition. I put my patients on two weeks of the quinolones (Cipro or Floxin rather than the Noroxin, which I use for simple urinary infection), followed by two weeks of the sulfonamides, and repeat the cycle three times. After twelve weeks a reduced dosage of the same medications is prescribed for as long as six to twelve months.

Chronic prostatitis has been likened to a fire in a haystack. The fire can appear to be out but continue to smolder underneath. The drug treatment has to be protracted. I continue with the drugs and the restrictions until the prostatic fluid is clear. It does happen, but not often. Frequently, the prostatic fluid will clear, but the patient will have a lingering malaise. At this point supportive psychotherapy becomes important.

I do not even object if the patient wants to try a little black magic – multivitamins or zinc, for example. The rationale for the use of zinc is based on the fact that there is more zinc in the prostate gland than in any other organ in the body. The thinking has been that if there is a problem in the prostate, there may be a need for this metal. What harm can there be in trying it? In fact there is scientific evidence that when there is a zinc deficiency, supplemental zinc administration will speed up healing. The zinc has to be administered by injection, though. There is no evidence that zinc in pill form has ever affected healing.

There is little place for surgery in the treatment of chronic bacterial prostatitis. Sometimes a patient will convince his doctor to resort to the knife, so desperate is his plight, but there is no assurance that an aggressive resection or even radical prostatectomy will rid a patient of his symptoms.

Besides chronic bacterial prostatitis, the terms "chronic non-bacterial prostatitis" and "prostatodynia" are used to describe prostate conditions. I am not certain if non-bacterial prostatitis is a separate illness or a bacterial disease in which the presence of bacteria cannot be demonstrated. Drs. William Costerton and Curtis Nickel from Queen's University, in Kingston, Ontario, have shown to my satisfaction that ordinary bacteria can hide under a "biofilm" within the prostate. I may be overtreating my patients, but I do not label them with a diagnosis of non-bacterial prostatitis without at least one trial of the antibacterials. Prostatodynia describes a painful disorder associated with anal muscular spasms. I treat these patients with muscle relaxants, anti-inflammatories, anti-spas-modics, and/or diazepam (Valium), but many cases continue to baffle me. I hope that one day hyperthermia – that is, micro-waving of the prostate – may prove worthwhile in the difficult cases. Covert bacteria that may escape anti-bacterial medications might be "cooked" by the heat. Hyperthermia has been tried for benign enlargement with unclear results, and its role in prostatitis is even more experimental.

Questions and Answers

- **How can my problem be in the prostate when I feel all the discomfort at the head of the penis?**

Branches of the pudental nerve go to the prostate and also to the head of the penis. When the prostate is irritated, it stim-ulates this nerve and the sensation is felt simultaneously at the head of the penis. This is similar to the way in which pain in the heart is felt in the shoulder tip because both are sup-plied by the same nerve. This process is called "referred pain."

- **If I keep having prostatitis, why can't my prostate just be cut out?**

Carving out the inner part of the prostate, as is done for benign enlargement, will leave behind an infected bed. Prostatitis will not be cured, the healing process will be pro-longed, and there is a high risk that a scar will close down the juncture between the bladder and the prostate. The only surgery that might help is total removal of the prostate, as is done when there is early cancer. In the past such surgery was seldom considered, because there was a 100 per cent risk of impotence and a 10 per cent risk of losing control over the bladder. The recent development of a method of radical prostatectomy that preserves potency and has a very low risk of incontinence may encourage doctors to reconsider surgical treatment for disabling chronic prostatitis.

- **Can prostatitis affect potency?**

At the height of the problem, all men are impotent or are anxious about their sexuality. They feel miserable and are often afraid, either that they will be impotent or that they will transmit the infection to their partner. When the symptoms have subsided, most men recover full potency. Some men report reduced potency, but it is difficult to know whether the problem is physical or psychological.

- **Can I give my partner a sexually transmitted disease if I have prostatitis?**

It is theoretically possible to transmit the bowel bacteria of prostatitis from one person to another through the semen. In practice this is seldom a problem, since there are not enough bacteria to cause an infection in the vagina. Nevertheless, I suggest using a condom for the first two weeks after the treatment has started. After two weeks, I think the condom is probably unnecessary. I have never yet had a man's partner come to me with an infection, but I must confess that I am not certain what is happening in the private lives of the people concerned.

- **If coffee is bad for me when I have prostatitis, can I use a de-caffeinated brand?**

Coffee contains over one hundred chemical ingredients, and

caffeine, per se, does not appear to be the only irritant. Tea, which contains caffeine, is much less of an irritant.

- **Why shouldn't I take twice as many pills as you have prescribed?**

It won't help. The chances of stomach and bowel upset would increase and the prognosis would not improve.

Concluding Remarks

It is remarkable that a gland that is normally so small, the size of a walnut, can be the source of so much male distress.

The capacity for orgasm is largely lost when the prostate gland is removed or diseased; benign enlargement can choke the flow of urine; cancer often defies early diagnosis and when advanced can kill; and infection is often impervious to anti-microbial treatment.

A prudent man will cut down on those items that appear to irritate the gland; namely, alcohol, coffee, and spices. He will drink more water, eat more fresh vegetables and fruit, and consume more fish and white poultry meat instead of red meat. He will submit to regular rectal examinations, the PSA blood test, and trans-rectal prostatic ultrasound exams when there is a hard area in the prostate, an asymmetry of the gland, or an elevated PSA reading. And he will maintain an active sex life.

5

Infertility

Infertility is, unfortunately, much more common than most people realize. Until this past decade, it was generally agreed that 10 to 15 per cent of all unions were barren. In other words, one out of every eight marriages was childless. However, figures reported in the last ten years (1985-1995) suggest that these numbers have doubled. And as the infertility problem appears to be more urban than rural, industrial pollutants and sexually transmitted organisms like chlamydia are presumed to be responsible.

Which partner is responsible for the infertility? In my experience, it is one-third male related, one-third female related, and one-third unknown. To find out which partner is infertile, exhaustive tests used to be carried out on the woman before the man was considered. This bias has been changing in recent years because investigation of the male is easier and less traumatic. There is no doubt that an infertility investigation should start with the man.

Investigating the Man

Infertility is a condition rather than a malady. Indeed, in most instances there are no other health problems – there is no urinary symptom, no sexual malfunction, no suggestion that anything else is wrong.

A person's medical history seldom yields any hints as to why there might be infertility. Mumps, if contracted after puberty, can destroy a testicle, but mumps usually affects only one testicle. An inguinal hernia repair can also choke the blood flow to the testicle, particularly if the repair is tight. I have seen a number of testicles damaged by hernia repair, but infertility is seldom a consequence, since surgery is normally done on only one side. And even when the surgery is bilateral, it is unusual for both sides to be injured. Certain chemicals, like lead, are known to be toxic to the testicles, but I have never seen a case of infertility attributable to chemical exposure. On the other hand, I have seen cases of testicular damage due to radiotherapy, or due to certain antibacterial drugs such as nitrofurantoin, which is prescribed for urinary tract infection. Damage due to drugs, however, is usually reversible after the drug is stopped.

The Physical Exam

There is one physical finding that a doctor looks for specifically: a varicose vein in the scrotum, usually on the left, called a varicocele. Ten per cent of the male population has a left-sided varicocele and, if there is no pain or discomfort, little fuss is made of it. But when there is an infertility problem the finding of a varicocele can be meaningful, because correction can improve fertility, as will be discussed on pages 116-18.

On rare occasions there can be a startling physical finding. For example, the vas deferens might be missing. This is the tube that conducts the sperm from the testicle to a storage depot. A man can be born without the vas. He can be fine in every other way, his testicles and hormone levels quite normal, and have no disability other than infertility. In effect, he has the equivalent of a vasectomy. It is not known why such a condition should occur. It is one of the possible consequences of stilboestrol, taken by the mother to control bleeding during pregnancy, but usually the mother's use of the drug cannot be verified, and stilboestrol is no longer prescribed for this purpose. So far we have no method to reverse this condition.

In other rare cases, the patient's testicles may appear extraordinarily small and perhaps a little firmer than usual. Furthermore, he may be lanky, with rather long arms. Such a combination suggests Klinefelter's syndrome, an aberration of the chromosomes associated with infertility. Another uncommon condition might be an absent testicle on one side and an apparent disorder in the remaining one. Another patient might have breast tissue more like that of a female, raising concern about testis cancer, or lumpy bumps along the vas, which is seen in tuberculosis. But the majority of men who come with an apparent infertility problem have completely normal sexual organs.

What is unusual is their tell-tale history: an active sex life, no contraceptive protection, no pregnancy.

Semenalysis

The critical test necessary to define the problem is semenalysis, an examination of the ejaculate. Different laboratories may offer different directions on how the specimen should be collected, but certain instructions are standard. There must be a three- to four-day period of abstinence from sex, the collection must be into a clean bottle, and it must be examined within two hours. Specimens collected into a condom or stored in a refrigerator cannot be interpreted.

The hospital laboratory where I work schedules men to come at pre-arranged dates, provides them with a container, and asks them to produce a specimen by masturbation. I was unaware of any problems with this routine until one patient complained to me of his ordeal. "I was thoroughly embarrassed. . . . You certainly did not prepare me. . . . Imagine, a young lady passes me a jar and tells me where the bathroom is located. The tiny closet toilet is ill kept and, in fact, not very private. I don't know whether those things affect the results or not, but I can tell you it was not a pleasant experience." I commiserated with him and acknowledged his complaint but insisted that when it comes to a hospital, modesty is left at the front door.

I have had to deal with patients who insisted that their religion did not allow them to masturbate, those who wanted to bring their wives and be provided with a place to copulate, and those who insisted on collecting the specimen at home and arrived with a jar containing a fluid-soaked condom. In general, however, semenalysis raises no more problems than any other laboratory test. As a rule, I request three separate analyses of the collected semen.

The detailed reports from the lab include volume, pH (degree of acidity or alkalinity), colour, presence or absence of fructose, bacteria, white blood cells, etc. All these aspects may be relevant, but what is most important is the number of active sperms per unit volume.

A specimen from a fertile man will show a high sperm count, over 50 million and up to 200 million per mL. More than 60 per cent of the sperm will have normal forms, not double-headed, tiny-headed, or giant-headed. And most of them will be vigorously swimming in a straight line. Specimens from an infertile man are likely to show less than 20 million sperm per mL, with many dead and abnormal forms and a lot swimming languidly in circles.

When no abnormality is detected in the semenalysis, and the patient is otherwise well, the investigation in the male partner stops right there. I advise the couple that I can detect nothing wrong and that investigation of the wife, if not under way, should commence.

When the semenalysis reports absence of fructose, it means that the man was born without the seminal vesicles. There is no corrective measure for this abnormality.

When the semenalysis detects sperm, but of a lesser count or vitality, blood tests for hormones are undertaken. The hormones tested are LH (luteinizing hormone), FSH (follicle stimulating hormone), testosterone, and sometimes prolactin.

Hormone Tests

If there is a problem with LH or testosterone, appropriate replacement therapy may help solve the problem. If the prolactin is abnormal, there may be a problem in the pituitary gland. But the most frequent finding is a very high reading of FSH, signalling irreversible damage to the testicles. I take the reading of the FSH seriously. The hormone is secreted by the pituitary gland in response to the number and vitality of the sperm produced by the testicles. If sperm production is proceeding normally, the FSH output is at a normal level. When there is no sperm or few sperm, the FSH level rises in response. If the FSH is high – two and a half to three times normal – I stop further investigation and counsel the patient that science has no solution for his condition at this time. If the FSH is normal and the ejaculate shows no sperm, I stick a tiny tuberculin needle into the structure located behind the testicle and suck out a drop of fluid into a saline-lined syringe. This tissue, which drains the sperm from the testicle, is called the epididymis. The drop is examined under a microscope and checked for the presence of sperm. If sperm are present, an exploration for a blockage is recommended. When the FSH is normal, I encourage the patient to keep his hopes up even if he is beginning to despair.

The test for hormone levels has made biopsy of the testis obsolete, as far as I am concerned. Testis biopsy is still being done, but I see no merit in it.

In the case of a man, the investigation for infertility is really quite simple. It takes no more than a few minutes to ask the pertinent questions, another few minutes to carry out the examination, and another moment for the tests.

Investigating the Woman

A woman concerned about infertility is seen by a gynecologist. Although I am not a gynecologist, I will try to explain what is involved.

During their reproductive years, women periodically shed the lining of the uterus, which has been prepared to accept a fertilized egg. This monthly process of shedding or bleeding is menstruation, and the cyclic occurrence is called the menstrual cycle. The entire process is controlled by the pituitary hormones LH (luteinizing hormone) and FSH (follicle stimulating hormone) working in harmony with estrogen and progesterone, hormones produced by the ovary.

When all systems are working normally, menstruation averages every twenty-eight days. During such a cycle, the egg is released from the ovary on the fourteenth day, and if intercourse takes place on or about that day, conception is possible. If menstruation is occurring every twenty-one days, the egg is still likely to be released about fourteen days before the beginning of the next menstruation. Thus, in all cases, the fertile period can be determined by counting backwards, and can only be guessed by counting forward.

When there is an infertility problem and the man is not the cause, the gynecologist does a number of tests.

He or she may scrape the lining of the uterus and give the scrapings to the pathologist to check the components of the "soil." Blood and urine samples may be taken at particular times of the menstrual cycle to check the level of the hormones. The Fallopian tubes may be checked for blockage by passing through gas or chemicals that can be X-rayed. The Fallopian tube normally accepts the egg released by the ovary and conducts it into the uterus. It is during this trip in the Fallopian tube that the egg becomes fertilized by the upward-swimming sperm. The fertilized egg normally descends into the uterus, but if it becomes embedded in the wall of the tube, the result is a life-threatening ectopic pregnancy. The Fallopian tube can expand only so far, and when that is exceeded, it ruptures.

The gynecologist may request daily temperature readings, because most women have a slight rise in their temperature when the egg is released from the ovary. Finally, the gynecologist may want to pass an instrument through the skin just under the belly button and into the abdomen to examine the ovary and, sometimes, to extract an egg about to be released. This test is called a laparoscopy.

It is thus apparent that investigating the woman for infertility is more injurious to the body than investigating the male, and that is why I recommend looking at the man first.

The Post-Coital Test

Some infertility experts will insist upon a post-coital test even before a regular semenalysis. The woman is asked to report immediately after intercourse. The ejaculate is suctioned out with the cervical mucus and examined. If all the sperm are dead or immobilized, a search can be launched for the cause, such as sperm-killing antibodies, particularly if the regular semenalysis has already been conducted and is normal. The timing of the post-coital test is critical; it is valid only if it is done during the woman's fertile period.

Treatment of Male Infertility

Often a man referred to me has a healthy partner and a normal medical history, physical, and semenalysis. Under these circumstances I recommend the following regime.

I encourage intercourse every three to four days. No more, no less. I point out that in different studies, largely on prisoner volunteers, sperm count was best when ejaculation took place every four days, and sperm vitality was best with ejaculation every three days.

At mid-cycle, when pregnancy might be possible, I advise the man to stay in his partner's vagina only for the first jet of ejaculate. After the first jet, the man withdraws. The first portion of the ejaculate is the most powerful, and the rest only dilutes it and reduces the chances of pregnancy. I also point out that if the frequency of intercourse is maintained at intervals of three to four days, during each menstrual cycle there can be no more than two or three chances for intercourse to be within forty-eight hours of ovulation.

I may ask the couple to have intercourse with condom protection for a six-month period. This is because, for reasons that may never be resolved, the woman may have developed antibodies that kill or immobilize sperm. Testing for this possibility is rather expensive and often inaccurate. When antibodies are found, the traditional treatment is for the man to wear a condom for six months to stop stimulation of more anti-body production, immunosuppression with cortisone, and inserting the ejaculate into the uterus with a syringe. These treatments are largely experimental, and successful outcomes have been few and far between.

Recently it has become fashionable to talk about "free radicals" and their suppression by "anti-oxidants," which remove oxygen from a chemical reaction and may thus counteract the action of the antibodies. The popular anti-oxidants are vitamin C, vitamin E, and beta carotene. I recommend a daily intake of 1000 mg of vitamin C, 400 mg of vitamin E, and 10,000 units of beta-carotene as good health promotion.

Tight underwear, particularly nylon bikini briefs, should be discarded in favour of loose cotton boxer shorts. The testicles are meant to hang loose, away from the body, so that they are maintained at a temperature 1.5°C (4°F) lower than body temperature. For similar reasons, hot baths and saunas should be avoided.

After doing all that, I suggest we wait one year and then meet again if pregnancy has not occurred.

Varicocele Ligation

When the semenalysis shows a low count, and when sperm are not moving vigorously, I hope to find a varicocele. If the distended vein is not immediately obvious, I try to induce it by asking the patient to force down as if straining for a bowel movement. The male anatomy is predisposed to the formation of a varicocele on the left testicle. The vein draining the left testicle empties into the renal vein, some 45 to 60 cm (1.5 to 2 feet) away. The column of blood appears to be too heavy for the one-way valves, and so destroys them. The result is a distended vein with incompetent valves – a varicocele. The problem is less likely on the right side because it drains lower into the *vena cava* (the main venous trunk). If the varicocele is present, or can be induced, surgical correction is recommended.

Surgery to correct a varicocele is a minor operation. It can be done on an out-patient basis, but I prefer to admit my patient. Under a regional or general anaesthetic, a 2.5 cm (1 inch) cut is made at the level of the prominence of the pelvic bone, about 2.5 cm (1 inch) from the margin of the bone. The muscles under the skin are split, the bowel envelope pushed away, and the swollen vein coming from the testicle identified. (Occasionally another vein nearby, called the inferior epigastric vein, can be mistaken for the testicular vein. The error can be prevented by tugging on the testicle – the testicular vein will move, the epigastric vein will not. This simple manoeuvre prevents accidental interruption of the wrong vein, something I have been called upon to correct a number of times.) A small segment of the testicular vein is removed. The wound is then closed. Patients admitted to hospital for the procedure can be discharged the following day.

Why a distended vein in only the left testicle should interfere with fertility, presumably a product of both testicles, is not clear. A long-standing varicocele does appear to shrivel the testicle. It has been argued that the extra amounts of warm blood passing through the distended vein heat up the testicle and cause the problem. Others have suggested that it is some waste product from the kidney or adrenal gland that would not normally get down to the testicle that does the harm. Such a factor has not been identified.

Nevertheless, this simple operation seems to improve sperm count and vitality. Different centres report successful pregnancy in 25 to 50 per cent of women who have partners with varicocele ligation.

The only other operation that might help overcome infertility is clearing a blockage, like a vasectomy reversal. This will be considered elsewhere.

Drug Treatment

Finally, if the sperm count is low but the FSH is normal, I try clomiphene citrate, a drug that stimulates greater release of FSH and LH from the pituitary gland. Half a pill, or 25 mg, is taken by mouth every day for approximately four months. If there is improvement in the sperm count, the drug is continued; if there is no substantial change, the drug is stopped.

I have not used any other drugs. Some experts feel that they can improve sperm count by administering testosterone for a period and then suddenly stopping. A rebound surge of sperm production is the hope. I am not convinced that it works or that it is free of potential harm. Gonadotropins (Pergonal), a drug prepared from the urine of post-menopausal women and containing FSH, and bromocriptine (Parlodel), which inhibits the release of prolactin, may have a place in the treatment, but I am not yet convinced that they have a role in male infertility, although their role in the female treatment is better established.

Treatment of Female Infertility

Some of the advice offered women, such as that offered men, has little basis in established scientific studies. The following are what I consider reasonable recommendations.

It is reasonable to ask women to lie flat on their backs for fifteen minutes or so after intercourse. This may help prevent spillage of the ejaculate.

If the post-coital test done at the right time suggests difficulty with sperm penetration, estrogen administered on days ten through fourteen may improve the permeability of the cervical mucus. Twenty micrograms of estradial (Estinyl) is considered an appropriate dosage.

If the egg is not being released from the ovary, there are a number of drugs that can aid ovulation:

1. Deltacortisone (Prednisone), at a dosage of 5 mg per day, reduces the male hormone level and helps induce ovulation.

2. Clomiphene citrate (Clomid) stimulates FSH production and thus can initiate ovulation. A 50 mg tablet is administered from day five to day nine. If ovulation does not occur, the dosage is doubled, tripled, or quadrupled. Occasionally there is overstimulation of the ovary resulting in multiple births. This is probably why this product is often called the super-fertility pill.

3. Pergonal is used when clomiphene citrate does not produce ovulation. Pergonal is FSH extracted from the urine of menopausal women. This is a very elaborate process and the drug is thus very expensive.

4. Bromocriptine is a drug that can be used when ovulation is inhibited by excess amounts of prolactin, a pituitary hormone that stimulates the breast to produce milk. Bromocriptine suppresses prolactin and thus helps induce ovulation. The elevated prolactin level may be due to a tumour in the pituitary gland, a problem that needs to be resolved as it may represent a life-threatening problem.

If the Fallopian tubes are blocked because of a previous tubal ligation, or from a stricture following an infection, it may be possible to unblock the system with microsurgery. In general, reversal of a tubal ligation is less successful than a reversal of a vasectomy. Infectious strictures are even more difficult to reverse. Often, rather than attempting to unblock the tubes, in-vitro fertilization (a test-tube baby) is considered.

Endometriosis

A large number of infertile women have a disease called endometriosis. It may account for 20 per cent of cases of female infertility.

Endometriosis is a peculiar condition in which tissue that normally lines the uterus is found elsewhere. The most frequent sites are the ovaries and peritoneal coverings of pelvic organs such as the Fallopian tubes and uterine ligaments, but it can be found in many other locations, such as the rectal wall, bladder wall, and ureter. This tissue behaves like uterine tissue, bleeding periodically, and, because it cannot drain out when it is located outside the uterus, is capable of promoting scarring. One theory holds that endometriosis is due to a backflow of menstrual blood through the tubes and into the abdominal cavity. But I have seen endometriosis involving the lining of the bladder, and it is difficult to explain how uterine lining can find its way into the bladder, raising questions about the theory. Furthermore, endometriosis has been found in the lung and in limb muscles and bones, sites even more difficult to explain.

Endometriosis is associated with painful menstruation and infertility. The condition is now treated with a drug called danazol (Cyclomen), which blocks FSH and LH production from the pituitary gland and, in effect, produces a temporary menopause. The treatment is continued for about six months and then discontinued. Menstruation returns after about a month or so, and in more than half the cases of endometriosis, fertility is restored.

Artificial Insemination

Artificial insemination means that the ejaculate is delivered to the vagina by means other than the penis. The semen can come from the woman's partner or from an anonymous donor.

If a man has a low sperm count, it seems logical to suggest storing his semen, perhaps concentrating it, and using it at the most appropriate moment. To date, however, all attempts to improve the quality of the sperm outside the body have not proven very successful. At some centres doctors have tried squirting relatively poor quality ejaculate directly into the uterus, bypassing the mucus at the cervix, which may be acting as a plug. The merit of this procedure has not yet been established.

"Sperm washing" techniques have become popular in recent years. The ejaculate is mixed with a fluid medium, spun in a centrifuge, and the surface fluid discarded. The remaining pellet is injected inside the uterus. In further refinements, another medium is added to the pellet, the mixture incubated for an hour, and the motile sperm that have migrated into the medium is used for insemination in what has been called the swim-up technique. When the medium contains albumin, the process is called the swim-down technique.

Artificial insemination of sperm from an anonymous donor is another story. Undoubtedly it works, and most centres report pregnancy at a rate of one in four attempts.

The facts are as follows. The man has an irreversible infer-tility problem. His partner is normal. The couple face a number of options. They might choose to accept their fate. They might give their name to an adoption agency. They might consider anonymous-donor artificial insemination. For many, it is not an easy choice to make.

I have encountered men who were for artificial insemination while their partners were not. Sometimes the woman is for it, and her partner is not. One man wanted to terminate the marriage to allow his wife a second chance at finding "fulfilment." The tearful wife would hear none of it. Another wife could not understand why her husband would not accept the idea of an anonymous donor. Sometimes the couple will try to trick me into taking sides.

Once the decision is made to proceed, further questions are raised. How successful is the procedure? One in four, as a rule. Any chance of malformations? Yes, but no more than in the population at large (in fact, according to reports, it is less). Who are the donors? Medical students, by and large, occasionally other university students. How carefully will the donor be matched with the husband? It is currently possible to match race, colour, and religion. Do you foresee any long-term problems? Only the chance of consanguinity, when the child by remote chance marries a close relative. Any other problems? There is a growing tendency among adopted children to search for their biological parents. Children who are products of anonymous semen might perhaps seek their biological fathers, if that ever became possible. What's my answer to that? I don't have any.

The anonymous-donor program has been severely curtailed by the AIDS epidemic. For medical-legal purposes, the donated sperm must now be frozen and stored while the donor is tested for antibodies to the HIV virus. Stored sperm is somewhat less effective, and HIV testing has discouraged donors.

The actual process of insemination is no more complicated than a routine pelvic examination. A speculum (what the gynecologist uses to examine the cervix and do a pap smear) is placed inside the woman's vagina, and the semen, which is in a syringe, is simply squirted against the cervix. Occasionally, if there is a problem with conception, the gynecologist may use clomiphene citrate to stimulate ovulation so that the insemination can be timed for a convenient date.

The Test-Tube Baby

Dr. Robert Edwards and Dr. Patrick Steptoe startled the scientific world when they announced that a little girl born in England in the summer of 1978 was conceived in a test tube. The mother's Fallopian tubes had been damaged beyond repair, but in every other way the parents were normal.

Test-tube babies are produced by a fine-tuning of science and nature. Doctors use a laparoscope (an instrument which is surgically inserted into the abdominal cavity just under the umbilicus in order to see and manipulate inside the abdominal cavity) to obtain eggs from the mother's ovary. The monthly release of the egg from the ovary can be timed exactly. Before it occurs, the ovary produces more and more estrogen, which is monitored by examining the estrogen in the urine. Just before ovulation there is a sudden increase in the level of LH and the woman is prepared for the laparoscopy.

When the ovary is examined at this moment, there are a few dark bubbles on the surface, each containing eggs. Using the laparoscope as a guide, the doctor passes a very long, thin needle through the abdominal wall and into a bubble, suctioning out the contents. Normally, the bubble would burst and the egg released would be captured by the free end of the Fallopian tube.

Sperm incubated in a special solution are then mixed with the egg. Different laboratories are reporting that no more than 35,000 sperm are necessary for fertilization to occur under these conditions. It should be stated, however, that 35,000 sperm from a fertile donor may be different from 35,000 sperm from an infertile donor. Nevertheless, fertilization by men with low sperm counts becomes a possibility, although most laboratories are hesitant to embark on this experiment because it is costly and less likely to be successful than when there is a normal sperm count.

The penetration of the sperm into the egg can be examined under a microscope. The nutrients are then changed, and, at the eight-cell stage, the embryo is placed inside the uterus.

The entire process is at the same time extraordinarily simple and extraordinarily complex. The pioneering efforts of Edwards and Steptoe have been duplicated by many laboratories around the world, but almost every centre will attest to a long trial-and-error period, and even today the process is in no way routine.

Furthermore, the concept of test-tube babies has opened up other possibilities. For example, the eight-cell embryos can be frozen and kept indefinitely. Not all embryos survive the freezing and thawing, but many do. It is also possible to use a surrogate mother, perhaps because the natural mother has lost her uterus or cannot tolerate a normal pregnancy. Or the mother may have lost her ovaries but has a normal uterus. Might she not "borrow" an egg, have it fertilized by her husband's sperm, and have the embryo implanted into her uterus?

The moral, ethical, and political quagmire created by legitimate scientific research staggers the imagination. I feel that our ethicists, lawyers, doctors, and politicians would be foolish to draw rigid rules, for what is right in one circumstance will be wrong in another. And the moral issues are not confined to the outer reaches of medical practice. I face it, for example, when a young man planning on getting married is referred to me for a fertility assessment.

"Why do you want a sperm count?" I ask.

"My fiancée and I feel it would be nice to know."

"Do you realize that the test cannot tell you if you will be a father or not."

"How so?"

"You may have a normal sperm count, but that does not guarantee a pregnancy. Worse, you may have a relatively low count, and if I report it to you, you might develop a potential problem that may never have occurred had the test never been done."

"You think I shouldn't have a sperm test?"

"I don't advise it. React to a medical problem, don't create one."

This advice seems to satisfy some patients. Others will insist on having the test done. Do I then give in, or do I tell them to seek someone else willing to do it? I am not sure I have resolved the dilemma in my own mind.

Recent technology originating in Belgium has made a one-sperm, one-egg pregnancy possible. The process is called intra-cytoplasmic sperm injection (ICSI). One sperm is captured by its tail, then injected by microsurgery into the centre of an egg cell. The technique thus bypasses the role of the kami-kaze sperm that prepare the way for the one sperm that actu-ally fertilizes the egg. I cannot say whether there are increased chances for foetal abnormalities, although the reports to date have not been alarming. Non-swimming sperm extracted from the head of the epididymis and traditionally felt to be inca-pable of creating a pregnancy have successfully fertilized eggs in this one-sperm, one-egg technology. Centres involved in these experimental trials have to charge for the attempts regardless of success. It costs thousands of dollars per attempt, and the success rate is about one in four. There is potential for unethical practices, although I am not aware of any.

Questions and Answers

- **Why does it take millions of sperm to create a pregnancy; I thought it took only one?**

Thousands, or hundreds of thousands, of sperm must bombard and eat through the wall of the egg before one sperm can actually penetrate. Research is being done on how the egg wall can be digested by other means, so that pregnancy may occur with fewer sperm. We do not know if tampering with the process whereby the wall of the egg is prepared for the penetration will result in deformed offspring or not.

- **My wife and I have children from our previous marriages. Why do we have an infertility problem now?**

There are several explanations. It may be because fertility is relative and declines with the years or because your particular male-female combination has created a fertility problem.

- **Since my problem is a low sperm count, why can't you store and then concentrate the sperm?**

I don't think that this question has been seriously examined by research scientists. On one hand, ejaculates of normal sperm are regularly frozen, stored, and used at a later date without significant loss of fertility. On the other hand, attempts to store, then concentrate, several sperm ejaculates appear to result in a substantial loss of viable sperm. Somehow, the two stories do not quite correspond. It should provide a promising area for research, and sperm washing and sperm manipulating techniques are becoming more and more popular.

- **When there is wide variation in the sperm count, is it a reflection of the person or the laboratory?**

Lab errors can play a role, but the more likely cause of the fluctuating count is the patient. We do not know why this occurs.

- **Can we do anything after intercourse to affect fertility?**

Some doctors instruct their female patients to lie flat on their backs for fifteen minutes after intercourse so that the sperm do not spill out. There is no scientific evidence that this increases the chances of pregnancy.

- **Why can't you use my sperm, even if it has a low count, and fertilize my wife's egg in a test tube?**

There is no reason why this cannot be tried. Most centres, however, want to restrict the technique to women with blocked Fallopian tubes, since there is a successful track record for this problem. It has not yet been established that test-tube fertilization can occur with ejaculate with a low sperm count.

- **If my wife and I were less anxious about it, would our fertility problem get better?**

The evidence that this is so is largely anecdotal. Stories of couples who became parents when they finally gave up the idea of ever conceiving a child are told again and again. What is not often related are stories of the many couples who remain childless after they give up.

There are studies that report that the sperm count of students is lower when they take exams. This is presumed to be due to fatigue, or caffeine consumption. But how fatigue, sudden illness, or fever can alter sperm count, when the production of sperm takes over seventy days, is not clear.

- **Is it possible for a person to be born with testicles but without sperm ducts (vas deferens)? Can anything be done about it?**

The vas deferens can be absent on one side or both. At present we have no way of substituting for, or creating, a sperm duct.

- **Can a testicle produce male hormones if it can't produce sperm?**

Yes. The male hormone, testosterone, is produced by Leydig cells, within the testicle. These cells are quite hardy. Sperm, on the other hand, is produced when cells lining a coiled and twisted tubule are transformed from stationary cells into mobile, tadpole-like units. The sperm-producing process is fragile, and the mechanism easily injured.

- **Are children born to couples with infertility problems likely to have birth abnormalities?**

There is no scientific evidence to support this fear. Indeed, the clinical impression is that miscarriages may be more frequent, but birth defects are less common.

6

Vasectomy
(and Vasectomy Reversal)

The Ethics of Vasectomy

Homo sapiens are very sexual creatures. No other animal delights in sexual intercourse the way we do. We respect no season, no time of day, no preordained frequency. I do not believe all of Freud's doctrines, but I do think he was right in suggesting sex as a driving force in our behaviour. But how are we to cope with the repercussions? Should respect for the sanctity of life be extended to every living sperm in the ejaculate? If not, why not? Should we respect the sanctity of the fertilized egg or embryo, or only the foetus when it is capable of life outside the uterus? Who can claim the authority to make these decisions?

I have no quarrel with patients and doctors who feel that sterilization contravenes their religious principles. I object only if they feel they must impose their convictions on others. Theirs is an arbitrary morality. This was clear to me when a blind man, already a father of two children, came to me after his parish priest had objected to his considering a vasectomy. I referred him to a younger priest who approved his request for a vasectomy without hesitation.

My only qualms about vasectomy occur when a young man requests it. Often he is unmarried but certain that he should not bring any children into this "ugly" world. I suggest that he reconsider, that a deep love might change his outlook. He may say that he is certain it will not, and that if I won't perform a vasectomy, he will simply find somebody who will. Is my conscience better served by refusing him, certain that he will be treated elsewhere? What I do is delay the decision and suggest we meet again in a year's time. If after that time the young man is still certain he should have a vasectomy, he will have no further argument from me. Some young men have returned a year later and had their operation. Some have not returned, and a few have come back to thank me for giving them the time to reconsider.

I have carried out a vasectomy on a severely neurologically damaged youth, supporting the request of his mother and his neurologist. I was not certain of its legality, so I called my Medical Association. There was no official guideline. I followed my conscience and carried out the procedure.

I have never done a sham vasectomy, as a colleague of mine once did. His patient's wife had become pregnant and the patient, assuming that his vasectomy had spontaneously reversed itself, asked for a repeat operation. A check of his ejaculate revealed no sperm. Rather than create a problem for "a nice couple," my friend elected to carry out a sham operation, cutting only the skin. He asked if I would have done the same. I said I would not have, but I had not been faced with his problem.

Normally I have no moral qualms about vasectomy. We do need some form of birth control. And in a stable domestic situation, when a couple feel they want no more children, vasectomy is the most reliable and least traumatic means.

The Operation

Male sterilization or vasectomy is the simplest "cutting" operation I do. I have carried out the procedure thousands of times in my office, and not once has a patient required hospitalization due to a complication. (I thought this record was broken after more than five thousand cases when one patient required hospitalization. The "complication" was actually an acute neurological disease called Guillain-Barre syndrome wherein various muscles become paralysed. My patient required artificial ventilation for a while because he just stopped breathing. Eventually he made a slow but full recovery. No one can say whether the vasectomy triggered the neurological disorder or not.) My secretary allots me twenty minutes for each case. This includes the time to answer questions, have the patient undress, disinfect the skin, and occasionally shave the upper scrotum when the patient has forgotten to come prepared as directed. Thus the actual time for surgery is closer to ten minutes.

At a refresher course for family physicians some years ago, I suggested that vasectomy can be carried out without the patient losing a drop of blood (certainly fewer than five drops), and without the use of stitches inside or outside. Two doctors in the audience were incredulous and asked if they could witness me at work. I told them they were welcome if my patients did not object. I can't recall now how well it went, or whether they saw one procedure or two, but I am certain that they were convinced.

My technique for vasectomy is as follows. First I disinfect the scrotum with providone-iodine (Proviodine) solution. Then I locate one of the vas and keep it fixed under the skin between my index finger and thumb. With my other hand I inject a local anaesthetic into the scrotum near my thumb tip, just on top of and on either side of the vas. Using a very small needle, I inject about 2 mL of a 1 per cent xylocaine solution and raise what looks like a mosquito bite. There is hardly any pain if the fluid is injected very slowly. A 3 mm (an eighth of an inch) cut is then made into the "mosquito bite." The anaesthetic works instantaneously, so there is no delay. A toothed forceps grasps the vas, and then for the first time the hand that has been securing the vas can let it go. A clamp with a curved and pointed end, known as a towel clip, is then looped around the vas. The surrounding thick outer cover of the vas is teased away, a 1 cm (.4 inches) length of vas excised, and the cut ends burned with needle-tipped electro-cautery. The procedure is then repeated on the other vas.

How much variation can there be for such a simple procedure? Surprisingly, quite a bit. Some doctors make a 2.5 to 5 cm (1 to 2 inch) cut in the middle of the scrotum. Why they consider such a big incision necessary is a mystery to me. Other doctors try to minimize the chance of a spontaneous reversal by looping back the cut end of the vas and fixing it in position with a stitch. But there is always the 1 in 400 to 500 possibility of spontaneous reversal after a vasectomy, no matter what technique is used. Looping may reduce the chance somewhat, but in my view the extra manipulation, with its increased risk of infection, is not worth the return. Some doctors cauterize the cut ends of the vas with saturated phenol, as is often done for the stump of the appendix after an appendectomy. This chemical cautery works well, but electro-cautery is simplest and, thus, best.

Another vasectomy variation, notorious for a short time, consisted of placing a gold pellet in the passage of the vas. The supposed advantage was that the doctor could reverse the procedure simply by removing the pellet. In fact this was not so, and the procedure is no longer popular.

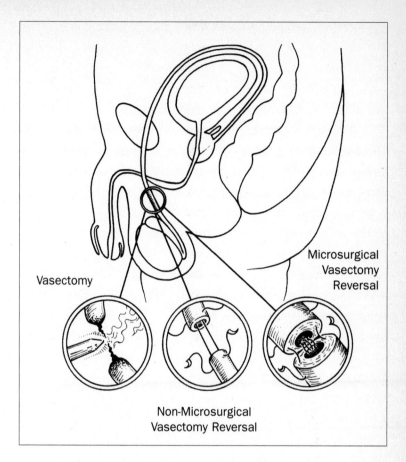

Vasectomy

Microsurgical
Vasectomy
Reversal

Non-Microsurgical
Vasectomy Reversal

Recently a no-scalpel vasectomy, originating in China, has been hailed as a major innovation. I have not attended the course offered nor purchased the instruments required, but for the life of me cannot find anything in the procedure that differs from what I have been doing for the past thirty years. It seems to me a reinvention of the wheel, that clever promotion has overtaken common sense.

I test for the presence of sperm in the ejaculate three months after the operation. I used to examine the ejaculate after two months, but found too many positive specimens at that time. Vasectomy cuts the sperm conduit between the testicles, where sperm is produced, and the ejaculatory duct. But the ejaculatory duct has to be totally evacuated to avoid conception. The number of post-vasectomy ejaculations necessary to ensure absolute evacuation has not been precisely calculated. Early reports suggested ten ejaculations, others suggested twenty, some thirty. A man who is sexually very active is more likely to clear his ejaculatory duct more quickly than a man who is less active. In general, a younger man has a negative specimen before an older man. Three months, though, is an appropriate time for the first check. If there is no sperm in the first ejaculate sample at this time, a second specimen is tested. I usually send my patients to an independent lab for the second check. Only then am I satisfied that the vasectomy has been successful. Even so, I warn my patients of the remote risk of spontaneous reversal and suggest a sperm test once a year.

I was sued once early in my career. After the first sample showed no sperm, the patient was advised to return for his second test. He thought better of it and returned only when his wife got pregnant. A sperm test then revealed copious numbers of sperm. He had had a spontaneous reversal. A second vasectomy was carried out without complications. Subsequently, I was served a subpoena. I went to court to make a formal statement but, fortunately for me, the case was dropped. The surgical consent form now in use specifies that the procedure cannot be guaranteed.

Other Methods of Birth Control

Most other methods of contraception are unhealthy or less reliable when compared to vasectomy.

In any given year, 25 per cent of the couples practising the rhythm method of contraception are faced with an unwanted pregnancy.

Condoms or diaphragms, with or without spermicidal jelly, are only slightly more reliable, with undesired pregnancy occurring 5 to 15 per cent of the time. Even so, these are perhaps the best methods of birth control short of vasectomy, which must be considered permanent.

The intrauterine device (IUD) is considered to be 98 per cent effective, but it has fallen into relative disfavour because of the risk of permanent infertility as well as the more immediate problems of pain, bleeding, and migration of the device. I know of one case where the IUD migrated into the abdomen. Problems with the IUD are uncommon but are alarming enough to have persuaded most pharmaceutical firms to discontinue the product.

The contraceptive pill may make pragmatic sense – it is, after all, 99.9 per cent effective – but it is so unsafe and unfair to women that I wonder why the women's movement has not made a bigger issue of it. When the pill was developed, it was tested on a vast number of female volunteers. It was then judged safe over many thousand menstrual cycles, implying that women could take the pill indefinitely. What was not clearly spelled out was that there was a difference between five thousand women testing the pill for three cycles and fifty women testing it for a lifetime, even though the two groups represented comparable numbers of menstrual cycles. Clots in the veins, strokes, and death caused by the pill came as a total surprise to the medical profession fifteen to seventeen years after the pill was put on the market. It can be stated today that the pill was never properly tested over time. It is argued that since complications occur in fewer than one in a thousand women on the pill, its use is justifiable. This may be so, except for the one woman who happens to be the unlucky statistic. Young women must decide whether the one-in-a-thousand chance of a clot in a deep vein, with its risk of a fatal clot to the lungs or the threefold increased risk of stroke, is worth it. The actual death rate attributable to the pill is 1.5 per 100,000 women between the age of twenty and thirty-five. Women not taking the pill have a death rate from a blood clot in the lung or brain of 0.2 per 100,000. Thus the pill increases the risk 7.5 times. Women over forty increase their chance of heart attack five times by taking the pill. Consequently, most concerned physicians will not allow women over forty, especially if they are overweight, smoke, have high blood pressure, or are diabetic, to take the pill. The risks are simply not acceptable.

Female sterilization, despite progress, is still a much more formidable undertaking than vasectomy. No matter what technique is employed, the peritoneal cavity has to be opened before the Fallopian tubes can be tied off. This means cutting through the front wall of the abdomen surgically or piercing the wall with a laparoscope to see inside the abdomen. The Fallopian tubes are clipped and the ends banded or electro-cauterized. There is always the risk of infection, which can become peritonitis (the collection of pus inside the abdomen, as in a ruptured appendix). A tubal ligation can only be safely carried out in a hospital operating room and almost always under general anaesthetic. And, just as with vasectomy, there is a 1 in 400 to 500 chance of a spontaneous reconnection.

What Can Go Wrong with Vasectomy

Vasectomy may be a simple office procedure, but it is not free of complications.

There can be internal bleeding, turning the scrotum black

and blue, hard, and painful. This can occur when there has been excessive probing and dissection by an inexperienced surgeon, or when the patient is too physically active in the first few days following the procedure. The scrotal sac is loose tissue. Thus when bleeding occurs it is not readily contained by the surrounding tissue and skin – there is space for blood to collect. A pressure-dressing or athletic support worn immediately after the operation may help, but the problem is best avoided by meticulous surgery and conservative post-surgical behaviour. I instruct my patients to lie low for forty-eight hours after a vasectomy. They can walk, but not jog or run. On the few occasions that a black-and-blue scrotum has occurred, the patients invariably confessed that they had not followed instructions. They had so little discomfort they thought they could chance playing hockey or football.

Another potential complication is wound infection, causing pain and fever. Internal bleeding and infection can occur together, usually reflecting poor surgical technique. Some doctors try to prevent infection by offering a course of antibiotics after the operation. This is not necessary and constitutes improper use of antibiotics. In the rare event that there is a wound infection, a broad spectrum antibiotic, such as tetracycline, is prescribed.

Perhaps an even greater surgical error is to confuse another tissue for the vas. I have heard a number of patients say that they have had an unsuccessful vasectomy. A second operation was necessary, they say, because of the possibility of a third vas. I have never seen a third vas and doubt that such a condition exists. It is a convenient excuse for the doctor. On the other hand, an absent vas on one or both sides is not so uncommon. This may be a rare complication of stilboestrol (a form of estrogen) taken by the mother during pregnancy.

Finally, as discussed before, the cut, tied, or cauterized ends of the vas may come together and the passage be re-established in spontaneous re-canalization. This can be due to improper surgical technique, but not necessarily. The possibility is 1 in 400 or 500 cases, and the risks are highest in the few months immediately after the operation but can occur at any time. I advise my patients to have a sperm test once a year, but not many follow the advice.

Unfounded Complications of Vasectomy

Some of the early objections to vasectomy were made by people who were philosophically opposed to the operation and sought scientific support for their stance. For example, it was suggested that 70 per cent of men with vasectomies would develop arthritis. At first glance the statistics were startling: 70 per cent of vasectomized men did indeed develop arthritis. But this percentage of the adult population normally develops arthritis, and vasectomized men are not more prone to the condition.

Another investigator found that vasectomized rats lost interest in sex, and the male hormone level in their bloodstream dropped to castrate levels. He sounded a warning to the human male population. But in rats, when the vas is cut, pressure builds up in the pipes behind the cut and the testicles are totally destroyed. In humans there is only a mild build-up of pressure and no damage to the testicles. This is one of the problems with animal research: some results obtained in one species are not transferable to another.

More recently, another reputable scientist found that vasectomy was associated with irrefutable evidence of accelerated atherosclerosis. Again, this was a finding peculiar to one species of monkeys and not substantiated in humans.

In 1993, reputable epidemiologists in Boston reported that men who had undergone a vasectomy were 60 per cent more likely to develop prostate cancer. Statistically speaking, this was a carefully done study. Indeed, the men who had not had a vasectomy had a 7 per cent prostate cancer rate compared to a 11 per cent rate in vasectomized men. This difference of 4 per cent represents a 60 per cent increase. But the Boston researchers did not account for all the variables in their study between those who had had a vasectomy and those who had not. And I believe that comparing men who choose vasectomy with men who do not, even if matched for age, income, education, and so on, is like comparing apples and oranges. In the first place, men who choose vasectomy may have a greater interest in sex, may, in fact, have higher testosterone levels. More importantly, other studies have failed to substantiate the connection between vasectomy and prostate cancer. Prostate cancer does affect 9 per cent of the male population, making it a very real problem, and if a causative factor linking vasectomy and prostate cancer is ever substantiated, I will abandon the procedure without hesitation.

Right now it can be concluded that vasectomy in the fertile man is safe, simple, and effective.

Vasectomy Reversal

Although the patient and his doctor undertake a vasectomy as an irreversible procedure, the patient's circumstances may change and there may be a need to consider a reversal. Sometimes the death of a wife or a child leads to a reconsideration, but the most common reason for reversal is the desire to have a child with a new partner. Sometimes the reasons are more bizarre. I remember one man whose Indian guru convinced him that he must be made whole. The psychiatrist to whom I referred the patient supported the request, so I proceeded with the surgery.

Unlike a vasectomy, the reversal is most often an in-hospital procedure, and there is considerable controversy among specialists about which technique to use. Imagine joining two spools of thread head-to-head and aligning the holes and you have visualized the surgical challenge of a vasectomy reversal. One school of experts firmly believes that microsurgical connections are essential for success, while another feels that the use of the microscope is overrated. I have done the procedure both with and without a microscope. When I use the microscope, the procedure tends to be more tedious and time-consuming. It is also exhausting. But there is an enormous sense of accomplishment at the end of the procedure, whereby several tiny stitches are used to join the inner walls of each cut end and several larger stitches to bring the thick outer walls together. When the microscope is not used, approximately four stitches right through the entire thick wall of the vas are used to bring the ends together. It seems to me that the results in both procedures are comparable and that the arguments about the technique simply shift the emphasis away from the real issue: how to test for the results.

There is no sure method to test the surgical repair. Fluids or dyes cannot be injected at one end to exit from the other. The presence of sperm implies a successful operation, but the quantity and quality of the sperm do not reflect the quality of the surgery performed. A high count does not necessarily mean a better sewing job, an inferior count does not mean poor surgery. There are other factors to contend with. For instance, higher counts are commonly expected when the interval between the vasectomy and the reversal is less than five years. Then again, although this expectation is firmly entrenched in the medical literature, some of the highest sperm counts I have seen after a reversal occurred after intervals of ten to fifteen years. Thus, the only important measure of success is a pregnancy. But centres that report 90 per cent pregnancy rates cannot prove that they have eliminated the "milkman" factor. Testing for paternity is theoretically possible, but does not seem appropriate in most circumstances.

Patients who request a vasectomy reversal are told that the success rate ranges from 50 per cent to 90 per cent. I suspect the first figure is more accurate.

Vasectomies and vasectomy reversals can present complications for the doctor as well. Six months after I had reversed a vasectomy, the patient returned to tell me that his wife was pregnant. I congratulated him but expressed surprise. Normally, I suggested, I don't bother to check the sperm count until nine to twelve months after the reversal because the results before that are usually disappointing. But if the wife was pregnant and everybody was happy, why not rejoice?

Some time later, my patient returned to tell me that his wife had left him and had taken the baby. He said that he recalled my implying that the baby might not be his, and that if such were the case, he was determined not to provide support. "Can you do some tests?" he asked.

I suggested that we do a sperm count. If the operation had not been successful, we would have laboratory evidence that he was not the father. The semenalysis showed more than a hundred million very motile sperm per mL – he was quite fertile. I imagined countless uncomfortable days in court.

But the patient returned to tell me not to worry. His former wife had confessed that he was not the father and told him that she would seek no support. There would be no lawsuits. Could he be considered for another vasectomy? he asked. I politely ushered him to the door.

Questions and Answers

- **Where does the sperm go after a vasectomy?**

Sperm live out their normal life span, die and disintegrate, and, within hours, cruising white blood cells swallow up the remains. There is no build-up of pressure, no discomfort, no danger.

- **Do you have to shave my scrotum to do a vasectomy?**

The cut is made into the hair-bearing portion of the upper scrotum. Unshaven, the hair is likely to obstruct the operation or find its way into the wound, like an ingrown toenail. What is now less certain is that shaving reduces the risk of wound infection. Indeed, a number of studies suggest that shaving the abdomen is associated with an increased rate of infection in the skin wound.

I ask my patients to come with the upper 2.5 cm (1 inch) square of the scrotum shaved on each side.

- **Will I need antibiotics or painkillers after the vasectomy?**

Antibiotics are unnecessary. On the rare occasion when an abscess forms, the pus should be cultured and an appropriate antibiotic prescribed. Strong narcotics are also unnecessary. A mild pain-killer such as acetaminophen (Tylenol or Atasol) may be used. Ice packs applied to the scrotum are probably the most effective method of controlling discomfort. Ice packs are easily made by placing ice cubes in a plastic bag and then covering the bag with a towel.

- **Can I get right back to normal afterwards?**

During the operation, if there is bleeding from the tiny veins that surround the vas, it is controlled by electro-cautery. If the patient is too active afterward, bleeding can restart at the points of cautery. Since this is better avoided than treated, it is best to keep a low profile for a few days.

- **How soon after can I have sexual intercourse?**

Wait two days, and then use your common sense. Hold off if there is any discomfort, but if there is no discomfort, it is up to you. Of course, until the ejaculate is clear of sperm, you must use a contraceptive.

- **Will my ejaculate be different in any way?**

The volume may be 1 to 5 per cent less, which is too small a change to notice. The colour, consistency, and odour are all unchanged.

- **Will the vasectomy affect my virility or my potency?**

Potency is largely a reflection of the testosterone level. Neither the production of testosterone, nor its release into the bloodstream, is altered by a vasectomy.

- **What about delayed complications of vasectomy, such as cancer?**

More than a generation (twenty-five years) has passed since this procedure was first performed, and millions of vasectomies have been performed throughout the world. Even in this large sample, no worrisome later complications have been recorded.

- **How soon after a vasectomy reversal can I become a father?**

Theoretically, the first live sperm can appear three months after a reversal, but live sperm in large numbers are seldom seen until a year after. I have seen counts that were low twelve months after reversal improve with the years. I have also seen high counts worsen over the years.

- **Is it possible that too much of the vas can be removed, making a reversal impossible?**

Gaps of 5 cm (2 inches) and more can be bridged. But with a large gap it takes more cutting of surrounding tissue before the two ends can be brought together, and the surgical trauma is greater. A vasectomy done close to the testicle is less likely to be successfully reversed than a vasectomy done a few centimetres away. This is because when the cut is near the epididymis, the far end of the vas must be connected to a tiny tubule within the epididymis, rather than to the other end of the vas. This microsurgery is less likely to be successful.

- **Why does vasectomy reversal not always work?**

There are a number of explanations. The technique may have been faulty or the testicles may not recover their capacity to produce sperm, or, if they recover, they may do so with less vigour. We do not know why certain testicles are unable to recover or what percentage of men will have this problem.

7

Scrotal Lumps

Scrotal lumps are easily detected, if looked for, because there is nothing but skin covering the structures underneath. An examination can lead to unnecessary panic when a lump is found, however. Let me emphasize that the vast majority of lumps are innocent. This chapter will discuss the various lumps that can arise, so that irrational, dumb decisions can be avoided.

It is common knowledge that a well-known British pop singer pads his groin to enhance his image and appeal. The story no longer sounds outlandish to me, as I have had a number of patients who decided not to remove their scrotal lumps because they wanted to look like "supermen." And back in the fifteenth and sixteenth centuries, it was popular for men to wear what is called a codpiece. This was a fortified bag or flap with a concealed opening in the front of men's breeches, designed to give the impression that the wearer was impressively well-endowed.

The modern equivalent is the athletic support containing a built-in metal cup to protect the testicles. As any man knows, the testicles are tender, delicate organs, with little protection from injury. Long ago, when it was less common to see female resident doctors, there was a female intern at the same hospital as I whose case history always contained the entry: "testes tender." We debated among ourselves which one of us male residents should enlighten her.

I remember one man who had a lump the size of an egg in his scrotum. When assured that the fluid-filled lump was not cancerous and could not become cancerous, he happily announced that he would pass it off as a third testicle. He'd already had considerable success with the ladies, he confessed. He'd just come to me to make sure he wasn't sitting on a cancer.

It was wise of him to see a doctor, because lumps in the scrotum are often benign but are sometimes cancerous.

Innocent Lumps
(Hernia, Hydrocele, and Others)

Innocent lumps include: hernia, hydrocele, varicocele, spermatocele, cyst of the epididymis, epididymitis, and mumps orchitis. Among all these benign scrotal lumps, there are two – the hernia and the hydrocele – that can reach enormous proportions.

Hernia

A hernia is a protrusion of an organ or part of an organ through a wall of the cavity in which it is normally contained. It is usually described in relation to its site or origin. Thus, there is a diaphragmatic hernia (hiatus hernia), which is the protrusion of the stomach upwards into the chest cavity; an umbilical hernia, in which the intestine or part of the intestine protrudes at the belly button; a ventral hernia, where a weakness in the anterior abdominal wall, usually after closure of a surgical opening of the abdomen, allows intestines to protrude; and inguinal hernias. There are three varieties of

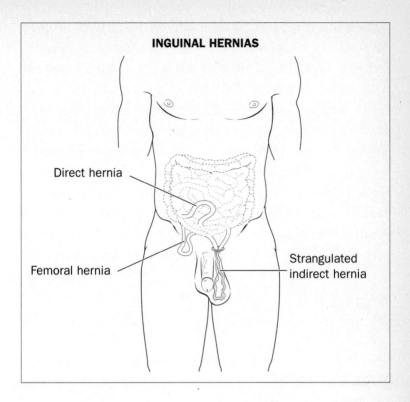

INGUINAL HERNIAS

Direct hernia

Femoral hernia

Strangulated indirect hernia

inguinal hernia: a protrusion of intestine at the groin because of a weak front wall is called a direct inguinal hernia; a protrusion of the gut into the groin where the leg meets the pelvis beside where the pulse of the artery can be felt is called a femoral hernia; and a protrusion of intestine through the passage taken by the testicle as it descended in the final month before birth to reach the scrotum is called an indirect inguinal hernia. It is the indirect inguinal hernia that can reach the size of a football.

A hernia is called "reducible" if the intestine can be pushed back into the abdomen, "incarcerated" if it cannot be pushed back, and "strangulated" if the blood flow to the intestine is cut off. This happens when the ring-like opening of the peritoneal tube chokes the bowel.

Some patients may choose to live with a hernia if there is no distress. Others may purchase a truss, which is a padded belt that works like the thumb in the dike, plugging the site where the hernia starts. The only cure for a hernia is surgical repair, which is mandatory when there is strangulation.

A hernia repair consists of pushing the intestine back into the cavity where it belongs, cutting off the hernia sac, which is the tongue-like protrusion of the abdominal wall lining, and repairing the opening and weakness in the wall that gave rise to the hernia. There are a number of techniques to do this. In principle, strong ligamentous tissues are sewn to solid tissues such as the lining of bone. When naturally occurring supporting tissue is unavailable, a synthetic-fibre material, like a Dacron mesh, is used to create the support.

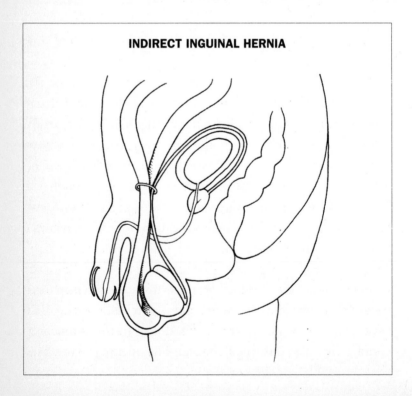

INDIRECT INGUINAL HERNIA

A completely new way of repairing a hernia has recently been introduced: the laparoscopic hernia repair. With the same instruments a surgeon uses to remove a diseased gall bladder through several portholes, the surgeon pulls back the gut and tacks in a patch where the hernia begins. The procedure has not yet stood the test of time, but the recovery period is remarkably reduced. I know one physician patient who was back to work within a week.

Hydrocele

If the peritoneal tube associated with the formation of a hernia is closed at the top but filled with fluid near the testicle, it is a hydrocele. Any man can potentially develop one. An injury to the scrotum or an irritation to the testicle can stimulate secretion of fluid from the cells that make the peritoneal tube. Such fluid will not disappear on its own. If the hydrocele is not large and doesn't cause distress, it can be left alone. When the collection of fluid is excessive (I have drained as much as 2.25 L [2 quarts]), there can be discomfort, even pain. The pale, clear, yellow fluid can be removed with a needle, but it will inevitably reaccumulate. If, after the fluid is removed, a scarring chemical is instilled, further reaccumulation can often be avoided. A commonly instilled chemical is the antibiotic tetracycline. Instillation of 250 mg of the drug dissolved in about 2 mL of a local anaesthetic is often, but not always, successful. In my experience more than 80 per cent have not required subsequent surgery.

Surgery for a hydrocele is very simple. The bulk of the hydrocele sac (peritoneal tube) is cut away, and what remains is turned inside out. Now the fluid-secreting surface is in contact with the inner skin of the scrotum and no longer in contact with the testicle. The scrotal tissue blots up any fluid that is secreted, unlike the testicular tissue, which could not

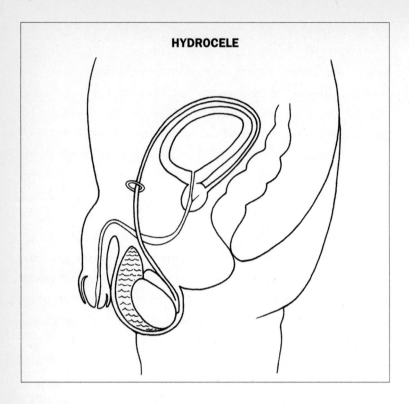

HYDROCELE

absorb fluid. An operation for a hydrocele can be done on an out-patient, but it is more common for the patient to be hospitalized for a day or two.

Varicocele

A varicocele is another benign lump that can occur in the scrotum. It is, simply, a collection of distended veins. Veins are part of the circulatory system that take blood back to the heart. There is no pump in the venous system that generates pressure as the heart muscle does in the arterial system. The venous system is a low-pressure system that depends on pressure from adjacent tissue, gravity, and the arrival of more blood to push the flow. Its flow toward the heart is prevented from

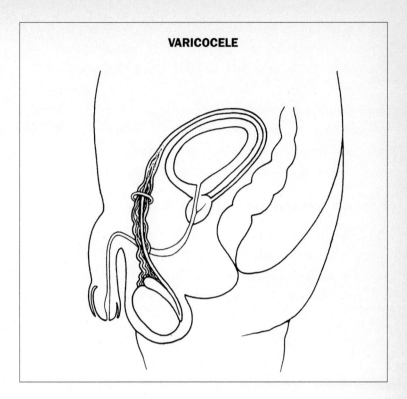

VARICOCELE

going backwards by a system of one-way flap valves. (You can demonstrate the presence of these valves in your own body by letting your arm dangle until the surface veins are filled with blood. Then, with your finger, milk the blood out of one vein, down toward your fingertip. Blood will refill the vein only to the point of a one-way valve.)

The veins draining the blood from the left testicle are particularly vulnerable to being overfilled. This is because the testicular vein empties far away (45 to 60 cm [1.5 to 2 feet]) and at a sharp right angle into the next vein. At least 1 per cent of the male population has a left-sided varicocele. The right side is less vulnerable because the right testicular vein drains lower down and obliquely into a larger vein.

It is simple to diagnose a varicocele. It feels as if there is a tangle of worms in the scrotum. This is because it is not one vein but a cluster of veins that has become distended.

A varicocele does not necessarily require surgery. It may be symptom-free, or the cause of only vague discomfort. Surgical correction is considered when there is considerable discomfort, or when there is an infertility problem with a low sperm count. (This is discussed further in Chapter 5.)

Spermatocele and Cyst of the Epididymis

A spermatocele is a fluid-filled lump that arises from the epididymis. How and why it occurs is not known. The epididymis is a conglomeration of tiny tubules directly behind the testicle, into which the sperm empty en route to the vas deferens.

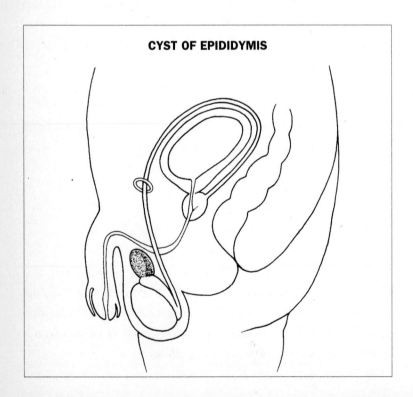

CYST OF EPIDIDYMIS

When a tubule blows up and fills with a milky fluid, often containing sperm, this is a spermatocele. The spherical lump can be as small as a pea, the size of a golf ball, or even larger. This blowout of a tubule need not totally block the passage of sperm, and even if it does, fertility is unaffected because the other side will still function normally. No noticeable change will be detected in the ejaculate because so little of the total volume of ejaculate comes from the epididymis.

A similar fluid-filled lump in about the same location behind and above the testicle can be filled with clear, colourless fluid. This is a cyst of the epididymis. Without examining the fluid, a doctor cannot distinguish between a spermatocele and a cyst of the epididymis.

Spermatoceles and cysts of the epididymis can be left alone unless there is discomfort. Surgery is a simple matter, requiring, at most, one day in hospital. The lump is approached directly through the scrotal skin and dissected off. It can often be removed as an intact sphere.

Inflammatory Swelling

There are three reasons why the contents of the scrotum swell due to inflammation:

1. bacterial infection (epididymitis)
2. viral infection (mumps orchitis)
3. twisting of the testicle (torsion).

Epididymitis

An epididymitis is an infection of the epididymis, the tiny structure behind the testicle into which the sperm exit from the testicle. The infecting micro-organism is most often a bowel bacteria, but it can also be chlamydia (a tiny bacteria that is transmitted sexually), a tubercle bacillus which causes tuberculosis, skin bacteria, or a virus. The micro-organisms enter the epididymis from the bloodstream or from the vas deferens. We do not know why bacteria in the bloodstream settle in the epididymis, but bacteria from the vas often flow back from an infection in the bladder, prostate, or urethra.

An attack of epididymitis can vary from a benign swelling with some tenderness to a feverish illness that is incapacitating. A mild case may clear up with oral antibiotics; in a severe case it is necessary to administer intravenous antibiotics and intravenous fluids. Bed rest, elevation of the scrotum, and application of ice packs are all part of the regime. Not too long ago, surgical drainage was carried out in severe cases, but today treatment using powerful antibiotics resolves the infection in most cases, and surgical drainage is seldom necessary. A severe case of epididymitis may extend into the testicle, causing it to swell and fill with pus.

Mumps Orchitis

Mumps is usually a childhood illness that attacks the parotid gland in front of the ear. When the infection occurs after puberty, there is a one-in-four chance of mumps occurring in the testicle in males and in the ovary in females. When the disease attacks the testicle, it causes a painful swelling whereupon the testicle may appear to be five times its normal size. Sometimes the pain is so severe that the nerve must be frozen with a local anaesthetic. Eventually the swelling subsides and leaves the organ a shrunken shadow of itself, the size of a marble, useless as a sperm producer and questionable as a hormone producer. Fortunately, the virus usually attacks only one side.

Torsion

Torsion is a problem that occurs almost exclusively in adolescent boys. It is not impossible, however, for the problem

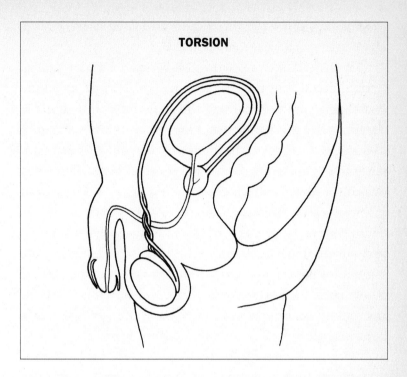

TORSION

to occur in older boys or men. In fact it is a wonder that torsion does not occur more often. As has been described, the testicle drops into the scrotum like a yo-yo on its string. The string or "cord" contains blood vessels and a drainage tube (vas deferens) and is wrapped in a spiralling muscle. When this muscle suddenly contracts, as in sexual excitement or in physical injury, the testicle may twist within the scrotum. If a doctor can see a patient in this situation promptly, he or she checks to see if the epididymis is outside its normal posterior position, and, if it is, the doctor can usually untwist the testicle manually and put it back in its normal position. But if the patient waits, it will be only a matter of hours before the tissue swells with fluid. The anatomical landmarks become obscured and make simple detorsion impossible. Surgery is often necessary to untwist the torsion, but after five to six hours of torsion, the testicle is unsalvageable and must be removed.

It is often difficult to distinguish between a torsion and an epididymitis. Lifting the scrotum is supposed to *lighten* the pain of an epididymitis and *worsen* the pain of a torsion, but it is unsafe to rely on such a test. Thus, when there is a chance that the problem might be a torsion, the patient is better off taken to the operating room. I have seen at least half a dozen missed torsions in my career. One such case was a medical student and the diagnosis was missed by my professor.

Sometimes surgery is carried out even though more than six hours have passed. The testicle is untwisted, bathed in a warm salt solution, and watched for several minutes. If there is any sign of life in the organ, a little pink hue, it is left in. At the same time, or at a subsequent date, the opposite side is fixed with three stitches so that it cannot twist.

Recently, the need to fix the opposite side has been questioned. One study suggested it was unnecessary, but because it was not conclusive, most urologists continue to fix the other side.

Cancer of the Testicle

In the Western world, in men between the ages of twenty and forty, cancer of the testicle is the third leading cause of death and the most common cause of death due to a cancer. Three new cases per 100,000 men are diagnosed every year.

It is prudent, then, for young men to learn to examine themselves for this cancer. The testicle should feel as smooth and as firm as a hard-boiled egg without its shell. Almost the entire surface of the testicle, except for a small area in the back where the epididymis attaches to it, can be examined through the thin scrotal skin. The examination is best accomplished in a warm bath or under the shower, with the testicle between the thumb and fingertips. A light touch with the fingertip is all that is necessary, since the testicle is delicate and sensitive, and any undue pressure applied to it will cause nauseating pain. An irregularity of the surface, or a firm lump within the organ, should be regarded with suspicion. (An irregular surface and hardness can also be due to chronic infection.) If there is any question of a possible abnormality, it should be checked by a physician.

An early cancer has no symptoms. Even when a tumour has totally replaced the testicle there may be no symptoms. On the other hand, a late cancer may be felt as a weight or a pulling sensation. Pain, caused by a bleeding into the tumour or a blockage of the blood flow within the testicle, may also be an indication of cancer.

An ultrasound examination is a very sensitive, reliable test to assess the state of the testicle. The pattern of the sound waves bounced off the testicle will be altered by a growth of just a millimetre in size. Ultrasound is more precise than a manual examination.

Cancer and the Undescended Testicle

The ultrasound test is particularly useful in men who have had surgery to bring down a testicle. Men born with an undescended testicle are twenty times more likely than the normal population to get testicular cancer. (Seven per cent of men who develop cancer of the testicle are born with an undescended testicle, and in 20 per cent of these cases, the cancer develops in the opposite, "normal" testicle.) Routine examination of this group of young men is often difficult, because the surgery to bring down the testicle may have created anatomical distortions. Ultrasound helps make the necessary diagnosis.

Classification of Cancer of the Testicle

Cancer of the testicle is classified as either germinal (arising from cells that produce sperm) or non-germinal (arising from any other cells). The non-germinal cancers are exceedingly rare and will, therefore, not be described.

Germinal tumours are categorized according to four different cell types:

1. seminoma
2. embryonal cell carcinoma
3. teratocarcinoma
4. choriocarcinoma.

These four cell types can occur in pure form or in various combinations. When the tumour is pure, seminoma has the best prognosis. The prognosis for teratocarcinoma and embryonal cell carcinoma is better than the prognosis for choriocarcinoma. Long ago, a doctor observed that when there is an element of seminoma in a mixed tumour, the outlook improves; when there is an element of choriocarcinoma, the prognosis is poorer.

Eighty-five per cent of teratocarcinoma and embryonal cell cancers secrete two measurable products into the bloodstream (alpha-fetoprotein or beta-HCG or both). These two "markers" are used to follow the progress of the disease and to assess the patient's response to different treatments.

Choriocarcinoma also secretes a specific hormone (the beta sub-unit of human chorionic gonadotropin – beta-HCG). The levels of this hormone can be measured and used to monitor the progressive stages of this disease.

On occasions, pure seminoma can also secrete these "markers," but we don't know why this occurs irregularly.

Staging the Tumour

Staging the tumour means defining the extent of the disease at the time of diagnosis. Testicular cancer is staged as follows:

Stage A. The tumour is confined to the testicle.

Stage B1. The tumour has spread to the lymph nodes but less than five nodes are involved and none is larger than 2 cm (.8 inches).

Stage B2. More than five nodes are involved or there is evidence of a node larger than 2 cm (.8 inches).

Stage B3. The lymph nodes are massive and can probably be detected by a manual examination of the abdomen, but there is no apparent spread above the diaphragm.

Stage C. The cancer is above the diaphragm or involves liver, lung, bone, or brain.

Management

When testicular cancer is diagnosed, blood is immediately drawn for the markers and the patient prepared for surgery. The testicle is removed through a groin incision similar to that used for a hernia repair. The testicle is simply pulled out of the scrotal sac by its cord. Radical removal is an exceedingly simple operation to perform.

While the pathologist studies the specimen, the patient is staged. A liver and bone scan, a lymphangiogram, and a CT scan are required to stage the disease. Liver and bone scans are discussed in the section on prostate cancer in Chapter 4. A lymphangiogram is an X-ray technique that identifies the size, number, and position of the lymph nodes. It is done with two dyes. First, a dark dye, injected between the patient's toes, shows up the lymphatic channels as a dark streak under the skin. A lymphatic channel can then be dissected free, threaded with a tiny plastic tube, and injected with another dye that shows up on X-ray. Subsequent X-rays show the size and distribution of the lymph nodes. The CT scan, a computer assisted X-ray, reveals lymph nodes larger than 2 cm (.8 inches).

A seminoma can almost always be cured with surgical removal of the testicle and radiotherapy to an area under the diaphragm, which is the site of lymph node drainage for the testicle. When the seminoma has spread to areas above the diaphragm, and the disease is extensive, chemotherapy is often used as well.

Teratocarcinoma and embryonal cell carcinoma often require lymph node dissection to stage the disease. But if there is no evidence of cancer beyond the testicle, lymph node dissection may be deferred. It is, however, necessary to follow up with CT scans and ultrasound examinations, and it must be understood that if ever there is evidence of nodal disease, chemotherapy must be started. If tests have already indicated that the disease has spread or that the lymph nodes are larger than 2 cm (.8 inches), lymph node dissection is also unnecessary, since chemotherapy is started right away. Chemotherapy is an exhausting and trying ordeal for the patient and cannot be undertaken as a preventive measure.

Choriocarcinoma can be monitored by testing for the presence of gonadotropin. In positive cases, chemotherapy is necessary and often succeeds in controlling what used to be a uniformly fatal disease.

Cancer in young people is totally devastating, and, as cancer of the testicle is not uncommon, I have seen my share of tragedies. Some patients handle their cruel fate extraordinarily well, while others come apart. Strong religious faith appears to help, but not always, since some patients turn against everything – friends, family, and faith. Several case histories are memorable.

A.C. was a twenty-eight-year-old senior medical student. While on a rotation in Boston, he noticed a hard lump in his right testicle. There was no pain, no urinary disturbance, not even a feeling of being unwell. He consulted the doctors at the Boston hospital, who all thought he needed immediate surgery. He elected to return home and came directly from the airport to see me. He was apologetic about disturbing me and, despite his apprehension, was calm and personable. He was going to make one fine physician. On examination, there was a stony lump in the body of the testicle, and there could be no doubt that the young man had cancer of the testicle.

I confessed my suspicion and we agreed to an immediate course of action that involved hospitalization, the drawing of blood for markers, and an immediate operation.

Removing the testicle was a simple fifteen-minute procedure. We looked for clues about the seriousness of the cancer at surgery. Did the tumour extend beyond the testicle? Was there a haemorrhage within the organ? We examined the testicle under the microscope.

In this case we got back the best report possible – the tumour was a pure seminoma. In fact seminoma is the most common form of this malignancy. It occurs in the widest age range, looks like fish flesh when cut open, and melts away under radiation. Its response to radiotherapy is so good that, even when there is no suspicion of a spread, a course of radiotherapy is offered.

A.C. was older than most students, having worked as a research lab technician before becoming a med student. He was married, too, but had put off starting a family until he had graduated from medical school.

I had his sperm banked and gave him the course of radio-therapy. There has been no recurrence of the disease. After graduation, he interned on the west coast. He became a father, with his frozen sperm, two years later. I'm curious to know if there is enough in the bank for another child. Theoretically, A.C.'s second child will be younger than the first in terms of the ovum, but just as old as the first as far as the sperm is concerned.

B.D., another memorable patient, was an angry young man by the time he came to see me. He had had a painful swelling in his left testicle for a month. The first consultant (Dr. X) had told him that he had epididymitis. He had been treated with antibiotics and told to cut down on his sex life, which the doctor implied was the causative factor. The second consultant (Dr. Y), seen just one week before he came to see me, told B.D. that he had cancer. He was seeing me for a second opinion. A quick examination of the scrotal content left little doubt in my mind.

"I don't like the looks of this," I said. "I'm afraid I have to agree with Dr. Y."

"Damn it," he said, "I'm twenty-six and I'm going to die."

"There's no need to be so pessimistic," I said, trying to be reassuring.

"But I didn't tell you, Doc, they also found something in my chest X-ray," the young man said.

I was furious with him. Why the hell hadn't he told me? Why was he wasting time getting opinions when he needed treatment. I was mad as hell, all right, but he sensed that a lot of my anger was directed, not at him, but at the disease.

"I'm not stupid," he said. "Do you see any point in chopping off my ball when the disease is already in my lung?"

I was taken aback. It is true that removal of the primary site when the disease has already spread may not affect prognosis.

"We need to know what kind of tumour it is so that we can offer appropriate treatment."

"Why don't you assume the worst and get on with the chemotherapy? That's what you guys want me to agree to, isn't it?"

"You know, you have a perfectly valid argument. In fact, if this were any other tumour, I might completely agree with you. You are concerned that cutting you up may spread the disease, that the surgery and the anaesthetic may weaken you, that the procedure may be more academic than therapeutic. But you're wrong! We need to know what kind of tumour you have. If you're lucky it will be a seminoma and you will respond to radiotherapy. If it's a chorio or an embryonal, you're going to need cyclical chemotherapy."

"Will you look after me?" he asked.

"You saw Dr. Y first, don't you think you should go back to him?"

"I don't like the way he reacted to my questions."

"You do have a way with questions," I said, and agreed to be his doctor.

The tumour turned out to be one of the nasty ones – an embryonal cell carcinoma that was already in his lungs. I consulted my oncologist friend (a doctor who specializes in cancer chemotherapy), and I visited while B.D. went through numerous courses of chemotherapy. He had the works: vinblastine (Velban), actinomycin-D (Cosmegen), bleomycin (Blenoxane), cis-platinum (Platinol), cyclophosphamide (Cytoxan), and doxorubicin (Adriamycin). His hair fell out. He retched and vomited, lost weight, looked cadaverous. Then he got better, put on weight, and raised false hopes. He died less than two years after his first visit. I remember our last conversation.

"Thanks, Doc," he whispered. "And I'm not mad at you because you talked me into submitting to your scalpel."

To this day I am upset that I did not have B.D. fully convinced that we had to have a tissue diagnosis. There was a chance things might have turned out differently – he was unlucky.

The drugs used in cancer chemotherapy are all poisonous to the human body. It is simply that they are slightly more poisonous to cancer cells than they are to most normal cells. Normal cells of the type that replace themselves rapidly (such as white blood cells, cells from the intestinal lining, and cells from the roots of the hair) are vulnerable to anti-cancer drugs. Thus, during chemotherapy, there is an increased risk of infection due to the depletion of the white blood cells. There is nausea, vomiting, and bleeding from the intestinal tract due to the excess shedding of cells. And because the cells of the hair roots are damaged, there is loss of hair.

The oncologist treads a fine line between killing cancer cells and preserving normal cells. His therapeutic objectives are usually achieved by using a combination of drugs in rotation. As experience increases, protocols for effective treatment are becoming more and more standardized.

R.M. was a thirty-four-year-old civil servant when I first met him. He had a charming and beautiful wife, a social worker by profession. They were an attractive couple, the kind you would expect to be surrounded by children. But they were childless. And not by choice.

R.M. had been born with undescended testicles on both

sides. At age five, both testicles were brought down, but there was a complication on the right side and the right testicle had been removed. Now the remaining, repositioned left testicle harboured a suspicious lump. The odds were that the lump was malignant.

After blood markers were drawn, the left testicle was removed. The pathology report indicated a teratocarcinoma, apparently confined to the testicle.

A lymph node dissection followed. This operation generally follows the finding of a tumour reported to be an embryonal cell carcinoma or a teratocarcinoma. The principle is that cancer spreads from the testicle into the draining lymph nodes before it seeds into other tissue, such as the lungs or liver. If we are able to remove the cancerous node or nodes, so the reasoning goes, we have a chance of arresting the disease before it seeds into other tissue. In reality, the disease has, with rare exceptions, already spread beyond the regional lymph nodes once it has invaded the nodes, and it may be that in most cases the lymph node dissection is an unnecessary trauma.

The lymph node dissection is a major assault on the body. The trunk is cut down the centre, from the level of the lower margin of the breast bone to the level of the pubic bone. The abdomen is opened and the entire contents pushed aside so that the posterior lining can be cut through. This is where the major blood vessels, the aorta and *vena cava*, lie. Both vessels and their branches are stripped of adherent fat and fibrous tissue which is intermixed with the lymph nodes. The operation has its share of complications. For one thing, stripping the artery strips the sympathetic nerve fibrils, and this results in a backflow of the semen into the bladder upon ejaculation.

Patients who are not subjected to the staging lymph node dissection are followed carefully and started on chemotherapy whenever there is a suggestion of a lump on ultrasound or on a CT scan, or if the blood markers are elevated. Elevated levels of alpha-fetoprotein are a sign that embryonal cell carcinoma cells or teratocarcinoma cells somewhere in the body are secreting the chemicals. Elevated levels of beta-HCG indicate the presence of live chorio-carcinoma cells. Certain seminoma cells secrete this hormone as well, however, which confuses the issue.

R.M. survived the lymph node dissection, and all his lymph nodes were free of disease. One year later, though, a 3 cm (1.2 inch) lump overlying the lower aorta was detected on ultrasound and confirmed by CT scan. Surgical exploration uncovered a node missed at the time of lymph node dissection. A course of chemotherapy was administered after the lump was removed. So far, four years later, R.M. remains free of detectable disease, but he lives with a sword of Damocles over his head.

One might wonder if it is not more logical to defer lymph node dissection in all cases and to proceed with chemotherapy at the first suggestion of nodal disease. Although chemotherapy may become the standard treatment, doctors who treat this disease in large numbers are not yet prepared to propose it. They point out, instead, that lymph node dissection has no major complications and appears to arrest progression of the cancer in acceptable numbers. They point out, in addition, that chemotherapy is not without hazards.

H.L. was a twenty-one-year-old engineering student when he first noticed that something was wrong. He started to develop breasts. Not the kind of fat that chubby boys acquire, but glandular, pubescent girl's breasts. His doctor referred him to an endocrinologist (a hormone specialist) who tested his blood and found the level of the beta human gonadotropin sky-high. He was sent to me with the presumptive diagnosis of a testicular tumour.

I examined H.L. thoroughly, but could find nothing wrong with his testicles. I called the endocrinologist and told him that I had found nothing.

"Are you sure?" he asked. "There's not much else that can cause that kind of reading. His HCG was beyond recording on the machine."

So we launched a head-to-toe examination and, finally, the diagnosis was made on ultrasound. A mass the size of a tennis ball was detected where the artery and vein of the right kidney are located. A CT scan confirmed the presence of the mass and, more importantly, detected no other mass.

At surgery, the lump dissected off the renal artery and vein very nicely, but it was attached to the *vena cava*. The vein, 3 cm (1.2 inches) in diameter, had to be clamped above and below the site of attachment. The "tennis ball" would not come off the *vena cava* without taking part of the vein wall. And no wonder. The tumour had extended through the wall of the vein and protruded inside the *vena cava*. If pieces of the tumour had not come off and seeded throughout the body, they were surely about to do so. When what remained of the *vena cava* was closed, the normal 3 cm were narrowed to pencil size. The student's recovery was remarkable. The HCG levels dropped dramatically. By the time the first course of chemotherapy was completed the markers were normal.

Six months later a repeat ultrasound study of the testicles found a tiny spot in his right testicle. The right testicle was removed. The pathologist could find only a microscopic scar, with no evidence of tumour cells, and we will never know if the removal was necessary or not. Undoubtedly, though, this was where the cancer started. Now, seven years later, the young man is alive and well.

I have described four cases from my practice. They were selected because each was memorable, but, in sum, they reflect the kind of optimism that pervades the field. Three out of the four patients are alive. Twenty years ago, after a diagnosis of choriocarcinoma, not one patient would have survived the year.

When there is talk about the "war against cancer," there is too much emphasis on failure – our failure to understand the cause, our failure to cure with surgery or radiotherapy or chemotherapy. We overlook the triumphs. Today we expect to cure 90 per cent of all cancers of the testicle. Progress in the treatment of cancer of the testicle, as well as in the control of leukaemia, lymphoma, and Hodgkin's disease, to name a few, are truly miraculous by any standards. When our society becomes more curious about the working conditions of under-funded researchers, we shall see greater progress. If a doctor is amply rewarded for restoring the health of one patient, how much more valuable is the work of scientists whose discoveries improve the health of the world?

Questions and Answers

- **Can I get a truss instead of having the hernia operation?**

A truss is a padded belt on a metal frame. It supports the weak area in the lower abdominal wall, through which the hernia protrudes. When it is fitted correctly and worn properly, it can control a relatively small hernia. On the other hand, I have seen men with a truss that is neither supporting the wall nor containing the hernia. Some men manage to avoid hernia repair for years by using a truss, but they are only dealing with the symptom. There is no cure for a hernia other than surgical repair. Since younger people are less likely to have complicating health problems, it is wise not to delay the operation too long. If a patient wishes to avoid or to postpone the surgery at any cost, and, if the hernia can readily be held in by a truss, there is no reason why it should not be tried.

- **Should I have my hernia repair with a local or a general anaesthetic?**

A local anaesthetic avoids the possible complications associated with a general anaesthetic, such as a pneumonia or a partially collapsed lung. On the other hand, if large amounts of the local anaesthetic are necessary, excess amounts may be absorbed into the body, creating cardiac irregularities. The fluid can also distort the anatomy and interfere with the repair.

- **Is it possible that my hydrocele will get better on its own?**

If the fluid is able to flow into the abdominal cavity, the hydrocele can disappear. This is known as a communicating hydrocele and is, unfortunately, uncommon.

- **Why does a varicocele cause distress in some men and not in others?**

A slowly developing varicocele will not cause any symptoms. A rapidly developing one will, but the degree of distress varies from person to person.

- **We've just found out that our fifteen-year-old has an undescended testicle. What should we do?**

Most experts advise removal and replacement of the testicle with a prosthesis. In cases in which the testicle is relatively low, however, and could easily be dropped to its proper position in the scrotum, I advise surgical correction rather than removal. It is necessary to follow the surgery with careful ultrasound testing for potential testicular cancer.

- **Why don't you do a biopsy before you remove a testicle only suspected of containing a cancer?**

On occasions when there is only a *suspicion* of cancer, the blood vessels going to and from the organ are first "soft-clamped" in the groin, the testicle is pulled out of the scrotum and through the wound, and a biopsy specimen obtained for frozen section examination. A biopsy that doesn't interrupt the blood-flow is never done, because it might spread cancer cells into the blood stream.

- **Is there any way to avoid going bald while undergoing chemotherapy?**

No, but it is certain that the hair will grow back.

- **Can a person die from chemotherapy for a testicular tumour?**

Yes, but it is unlikely. The cancer is a far greater threat to life, and there is no doubt that chemotherapy cures the vast majority of patients with testicular cancers.

- Can a person regain fertility after a course of chemotherapy?

It is possible, but cannot be predicted. Sperm-banking, when
possible, is the best precaution.

- Does a man lose his potency after chemotherapy?

It is possible, but not likely. The testosterone-producing cells
of the testicle are not easily damaged. A temporary state of
impotence can result from the weakened condition.

8

Sex and Sex Changes

Human sexuality is the stuff of poems, songs, fantasy, and much befuddlement. I can't pretend to be an expert on the delicate or delicious aspects of sexuality, but I can review what we know about the stages of human sexual growth, beginning by describing the basic element of human sexuality: the chromosome.

Chromosomes

Chromosomes are the genetic blueprint of human beings. They define each person's sex and biological potential. Half come from the father and half from the mother. The human species has twenty-three pairs of chromosomes, including one pair of sex chromosomes, which determine gender. The father may contribute either an X or a Y chromosome, the mother always contributes an X chromosome. When an X chromosome comes from the father, and combines with an X chromosome of the mother, it creates an XX sex chromosome pattern in the infant, and the baby is a genetic female. When the father contributes a Y chromosome, the resulting XY pattern produces a genetic male. The father's chromosome, therefore, determines the sex of the child.

The Y chromosome causes the inner part of the primitive sex organ to become the testicles. These early testicles produce testosterone, which in turn stimulates the appropriate primitive tissue to become the various male sex organs. In rare cases, when the male hormone is not available, even though there is an XY chromosome pattern, the baby will not develop male sex organs and will have the outward appearance of a girl. When the male hormone level is elevated, even a girl baby will show more male features, such as an enlarged clitoris. When there are two X chromosomes, the outer parts of the primitive gonads become the ovaries, and the baby develops both the internal and external sex organs of a girl.

Sometimes there is an irregularity in the inherited pattern of the sex chromosomes, as, for example, in Klinefelter's syndrome and Turner's syndrome. In Klinefelter's syndrome, the infant inherits an extra chromosome, ending up with an XXY pattern. This irregularity produces lanky arms, excess breast development, a penis with small testicles and no sperm. In Turner's syndrome the infant is missing a sex chromosome, ending up with an XO pattern. This person will look like a girl but will often be very short, with something like the webbing in a frog's foot on each side of the neck, no breasts, and non-functional ovaries.

Other bizarre patterns of chromosomal inheritance, associated with infertility and frequent mental retardation, do exist, but these are rare. Most of us are born with straightforward XX or XY sex chromosomes. We are boys or girls. We may be infinitely various, but we will have a common evolutionary development – from child, to adolescent, to adult, and, perhaps, to parenthood. And our first sex change will be that of puberty.

Puberty

The process of puberty, the first "sex change," is different for boys and girls, but in each case there are predictable physical changes.

Puberty in Girls

First there is a growth spurt, usually around age twelve. Breast development may start as early as age eight or as late as age thirteen, and even later on occasion. Pubic hair usually appears before menstruation, which, on the average, begins at age thirteen. All changes evolve gradually. The breasts, for example, start to bud. Then the pigmented area surrounding the nipple enlarges. Next, the entire breast increases in size, the nipple and pigmented areas bulge, and, finally, the breast assumes its fully rounded, adult appearance. Pubic hair changes from straight, sparse, and lightly pigmented, to curly, coarser, pigmented hair in the shape of a triangle pointing down. Menstruation is irregular at first, and may not always be associated with ovulation.

Puberty in Boys

A boy's growth spurt usually occurs around age fourteen, but in boys the changes of puberty occur over a wider age range than they do in girls. Boys experience a voice change, a deepening due to the thickening of the vocal cords. Facial hair begins to grow. Muscle development increases. The scrotum, testicles, and penis gradually enlarge, and pubic hair appears, becomes thicker, and looks like a triangle pointing to the belly button. Also, 50 per cent of all boys experience a breast enlargement which recedes within two years. All changes occur gradually over a two- to three-year period. The first ejaculation at about age fourteen is usually from masturbation or from nocturnal emission.

Virginity

The loss of virginity and the beginning of an active sex life may be considered the next sex change. In boys, there are no physical changes associated with the loss of virginity. In girls, the hymen may be torn. Some people and certain societies place great emphasis on this change. In fact the hymen is a rim of very ordinary tissue. I have been asked a number of times to reconstitute a torn hymen to simulate virginity. Although I have never carried out the procedure, gynecologists who do tell me that "virginity" is restored by stitching together the torn remnants of the hymen. To prevent unyielding scar tissue, the operation must be timed so that the hymen will be torn again a few days later.

The Average Sex Life

It is presumptuous to suggest that there is a "normal" sex life. Just as in exercise, diet, or fashion, what is right for one individual may be too much, or too little, for another. Nevertheless, there are surveys on the frequency of ejaculation within the life cycle, and statements regarding national "averages" can be made.

There is little doubt that, on the average, men in their early twenties have more ejaculations than at any other time of their lives. Women, generally, experience their strongest sex drive and most frequent orgasms in their late thirties. For men, the average frequency of ejaculation per week during the twenties is four to five times; two to four during the thirties;

once or twice during the forties; none to once a week during the fifties. From the sixties on, frequency is most often expressed per month, and once or twice is the usual frequency quoted. In one survey, two-thirds of men in their sixties were sexually active, as were one-third of men in their seventies. Of course, sexual activity is defined in these studies only as ejaculation, and many older people (to say nothing of gay women) consider this too narrow a definition of sexuality.

There is no doubt that men over the age of sixty take longer to achieve an erection, require more direct penile stimulation, have decreased firmness, and may experience less intensity with ejaculation. Also, after ejaculation a longer time is necessary to reacquire an erection. But orgasms can be felt, even without ejaculation, and orgasms that are less intense may be totally sexually fulfilling. There is no question that, with age, the frequency of sexual activity wanes, but not necessarily the sexual pleasure.

At any rate, I don't pay much attention to the "normal" figures. Often, when I provide them to patients, they happily conclude that their sexuality is livelier than the reported averages. And my advice to an older man who wants to know why he isn't performing as frequently as his boasting neighbour is borrowed from a cartoon I once saw: "Well, no reason why you can't say the same thing."

The Female Menopause

Excluding childbirth, the menopause is the next major sexual change in women, and although it is a very important stage of a woman's life, most men know almost nothing about it.

Menopause is signalled by the cessation of menstruation. This occurs at about age fifty, but there is a wide age variation.

As a rule, it is true that the earlier a woman begins to menstruate, the later she will finish.

Some women have no noticeable symptoms associated with menopause, yet others report symptoms such as diminished vaginal lubrication, irritation with urination, increased irritability, and depression. Two out of three women get hot flashes, which they describe as a sudden feeling of heat or redness in the face and upper body that lasts for several minutes. The hot flashes can recur for one to five years.

Women who have a difficult menopause need their partner's understanding and support. Menopause is not a made-up or psychological disturbance – it is physiologically based. Most of the undesirable symptoms of menopause are attributable to a lack of estrogen, a hormone normally produced by the ovaries. We do not know why the ovaries produce less or no estrogen in middle age, but they do.

Menopausal symptoms and disorders can all be alleviated by the administration of estrogen. Changes in the skin, such as wrinkling and thinning, can be slowed down. Bone weakening, or osteoporosis, can be diminished, especially when combined with an adequate dietary intake of calcium. Vaginal and bladder infections also become less frequent.

But estrogen-replacement therapy increases the risk of cancer of the uterine lining. The normal incidence is one in a thousand per year. When estrogen is administered, the risk is increased four times.

You might advise your partner that today gynecologists use a combination of estrogen and progesterone. This mixture most closely resembles normal female physiology and so does not have the risks of estrogen alone. A number of studies have now confirmed that cancer of the uterine lining does not occur with any increased frequency in women treated with both hormones. But with the estrogen-progesterone combination, a woman still has her menstrual bleeding, and this consequence may deter some women.

If your partner has disagreeable menopausal symptoms, and if she has had a hysterectomy, I suggest estrogen replacement. If your partner wants treatment and still has her uterus, I would suggest a combination of estrogen and progesterone.

Some women will want treatment and others will not. In either case there is no diminishing of sexual desire due to menopause, and logistical problems, such as a lack of lubrication, should they occur, can be treated. By all means continue sexual activity.

The Male Menopause

The male menopause, or climacteric, is, perhaps, more an intriguing concept than a scientific fact. It is defined in terms of a collection of symptoms: listlessness, poor appetite, weight loss, impaired ability to concentrate, weakness, irritability, depressed libido, and depressed erections. There is nothing very specific about these symptoms; a man complaining of any or all of them could just as easily have anaemia, depression, or an undiagnosed malignancy.

If there were a male counterpart to female menopause, we should be able to demonstrate rather sudden lowered levels of circulating testosterone and a corresponding elevation in the pituitary gonadotropins at a particular period in life. The pattern that has been noted instead is a slow, gradual lowering of the testosterone level and an uneven loss of testicular tissue. Elderly men, even in their eighties and nineties, still have some testicular function, which explains why they can become fathers. Charlie Chaplin may be the most famous over-seventy-year-old father, but he is by no means the only one.

Male menopause is an intriguing concept, but not a likely reality. It is perhaps more to the point to look at stress and pressure as causes of unpleasant male mid-life symptoms than to believe in this ethereal concept.

Like changes in fashion, enthusiasm for the concept of male menopause waxes and wanes. Recently there has been a revival of interest in Britain, coincident with the release of an oral male hormone preparation called testosterone unde-canoate (Andriol). The usual male hormone, testosterone, prepared for oral use can damage the liver. Andriol, it is claimed, is safer. A 40 mg tablet taken three times a day can substitute for inadequate production of testosterone. I have little experience with the product, but I do know it to be con-siderably more expensive than testosterone used as an intra-muscular injection.

Manipulated Sex Change

Admittedly, sexuality is a complex subject, and giving medical advice becomes more complicated when the disorder is psy-chological rather than physical. In these androgynous times, external appearances are often not enough to distinguish gender. Neither, even, are chromosomes if a person does not feel comfortable with his or her given sex. But science, undaunted, has developed a quantifiable way to assess gender.

Whether a person is male or female is medically defined in five ways:

1. whether the person has male or female chromosomes;
2. whether the person has male or female internal sex organs (testicles, prostate, and seminal vesicles in men; ovaries, Fallopian tubes, uterus, cervix, and vagina in women);
3. in terms of the external sex organs (penis and scrotum in

men; labia majora, labia minora, clitoris, and breasts in
women);

4. in terms of the psyche;
5. in terms of how the infant was raised – whether as a boy or
a girl.

Studies show that of these five criteria, the most important psychologically is how the infant was raised. Thus, if a
boy was accidentally, or deliberately, brought up as a girl,
despite having external and internal male characteristics, he
may feel himself to be a girl. In some cases, a person's sense of
identity will best be served by altering his or her external
appearance to that of the opposite sex. In many other cultures
and in ancient civilizations, sex change was simply accomplished by donning the attire and taking on the demeanour of
the other sex. Since the 1950s, doctors have become involved
in sex-change manipulation and now sex-change surgery is
modern society's way of dealing with transsexuals.

The Sex-Change Operations

Male-to-Female

A male transsexual is one who feels he was born with the
wrong sex. He is different from a male transvestite, who dresses
in women's clothing for sexual arousal, or a male homosexual,
who prefers sexual relations with another male. The true
transsexual wishes to alter himself physically, to actually attain
what he deeply feels is his real sexual identity. This means he
must have a sex-change operation. Often a psychiatric assessment as to whether or not the applicant is a true transsexual
is required before an operation is allowed. And, on rare occasions, even the psychiatrist is fooled by someone who is not
really a transsexual but believes a sex change will solve certain

problems. There is a bond among the transsexual population, and they may well discuss their pre-op interviews – what was asked and what the response should be.

Once a person is categorized as a true transsexual, treatment begins. First, the female hormone estrogen is taken by mouth. Electrolysis removes unwanted hair and, sometimes, breasts are augmented by plastic surgery. This process of outward feminization can take up to two years. An operation to alter the external genitalia is then carried out.

A number of surgical techniques have been devised to create outer lips and a vagina. One procedure involves taking a short segment of large bowel and making it into a vagina. In another, a free skin graft is wrapped around a tubing to make a vagina. Possibly the most ingenious technique, which I will describe below, utilizes the skin of the penis to form the vagina – a procedure that seems, to me, to make the most sense.

After the patient is under a general anaesthetic, the legs are placed in stirrups and the body positioned as if for a prostate operation or delivery of a baby. A catheter is inserted in the tip of the penis, through the urethra, and into the bladder. A cut is made around the circumference of the penis near the head. The skin covering the shaft of the penis is pushed down toward the body. The inside tissue, now bare, is removed carefully without damaging the urethra. The external skin of the penis is then pulled up and pushed back in on itself to make a vagina. This inverted skin still has to be brought down below the pubic bone to be in the proper position, and this is done by cutting and pulling. Some of the scrotal skin is used to fashion what will resemble the outer lips, and the excess is discarded. The carefully preserved urethra, sticking up with its catheter in the centre of the new vagina, is then amputated at an appropriate length. It is pulled through a buttonhole opening made in the vagina and stitched in place.

Since skin has a natural tendency to contract, however, surgically constructed vaginas tend to close down. This is counteracted by plastic moulds of varying sizes that are used to dilate the vagina and maintain the appropriate size. Daily dilatation is mandatory at first. Eventually, finger dilatation is sufficient to maintain adequate vaginal size.

There are a number of complications associated with the male-to-female sex-change operation. Immediate complications include internal blood collection, wound infection, infection of the pubic bone, or a hole between the urethra and the vagina. Delayed complications include narrowing where the urethra was sewn to the skin, urinary tract infection, prostatitis, or closing down of the vagina.

The results can also be cosmetically undesirable: the scrotal labia may be too scanty or too redundant; the urinary opening may be placed too high, causing havoc with urination; the labia and the vagina may be poorly aligned. Finally, even when the results are pleasing to the surgeon, they may not live up to the expectations of the patient.

Female-to-Male

Fewer women than men are openly transsexual. It may be, however, that the transsexual problem occurs with equal frequency in the sexes but remains more covert with women. Perhaps women realize that the surgical challenge is more difficult and more likely to fail in the female-to-male conversion.

To date, doctors have attempted to fashion a penis from tubed flaps taken from the abdomen and to fashion a scrotum from the labia. Creating a continuous urinary channel from the natural opening through the new penis has proven a formidable task. And, even with the implantation of a penile and testicular prosthesis, there is no sexual sensation in the surgically constructed penis. Most centres have abandoned this sex-change operation.

I have encountered a number of transsexuals in my practice, but I have never done a sex-change operation. The hospital where I work has decided not to become involved with this health problem, and its stance is not unique. The hospital argues that a success rate of one in three is not good enough, that there is an alarming rate of suicide, depression, and psychosis, even after successful surgery, and that its budget is stretched to the limit.

A friend of mine who used to do sex-change operations at another hospital has abandoned doing them. He says he couldn't handle the constant calls, the veiled threats, the persistent complaints.

I have had some interesting encounters with the transsexual population. I remember asking a patient, who was waiting to have his procedure done in New York, how he would manage to find the funds to pay for the operation.

"I work as a prostitute," he replied.

I was baffled and showed it. Estrogen had given him the body contours of a female and, with make-up and a dress, he could easily pass for a nice-looking woman. But he still had a penis, scrotum, and testicles.

"Oh, I warn my customers," he said. "Some men are turned off, but most of the clients are curious to know what I can offer."

One transsexual wanted her surgery revised. I examined her and was most impressed with the cosmetic results. And I told her so.

"What could be the matter?" I asked.

"He didn't chop enough off," she said. "When I make love, I still get an erection, and it hurts me and it hurts my partner."

I told her that she was lucky, that next time she could end up with an infection, internal bleeding, or narrowing of the opening.

"But I can't go on like this, it hurts too much," she pleaded. So we arranged a revision. But after she cancelled twice, I was not displeased that the surgery might never come to pass. Now, many years have passed since we agreed to the surgery, and it has never happened.

Another transsexual needed a revision where the vagina made of large bowel met the skin. The opening was so small it did not allow evacuation of mucus. She had revision surgery with satisfactory results that allowed her to resume sex. A few years later she choked on a chicken bone and died. She was my first transsexual patient and the source of many others. Since her death I have not seen any new transsexual patient.

Sex changes in average, everyday life are complicated enough to deal with. I do not envy the transsexual who feels trapped inside the wrong sex. Neither do I envy the surgeon who attempts to make the transsexual's flesh correspond to a psychic need.

Questions and Answers

• **Can my partner be allergic to my sperm?**

It is uncommon but possible. I treated one woman who broke out in hives whenever her husband didn't use a condom. An immuno-chemist was very interested in investigating what component in the semen made her allergic, but, once the hives were cured by an antihistamine pill, taken orally before sex, the patient left the study.

- **Is it possible that my penis is shrivelling up and disappearing?**

The penis can become smaller when the male hormone level drops to castrate level, such as after surgical removal of the testicles. More often, however, the "shrinkage" of the penis is simply an overgrowth of adjacent fat tissue, and more apparent than real.

- **Can an amputated penis be sewn back on?**

Delicate microsurgery can rejoin an amputated penis, but erection will not reoccur unless the nerve is rejoined as well. This task is more formidable. Besides the Bobbitt case, which got wide publicity, there have been a number of other instances of penis reattachments. I recall one that was done in the hospital in which I work. Microsurgical connections of the artery and nerve were carried out by plastic surgeons. I know the cosmetic results were acceptable, but I am not sure whether erections have returned.

- **Why do people have such a negative attitude about masturbation?**

There is a strong tradition in Western civilization condemning pleasure without purpose. Such pleasure is even said to contravene the will of God. Medical science has known for some time that masturbation causes no bodily or psychological harm, but only in recent years has it publicized this fact.

- **Should all menopausal or post-menopausal women take replacement hormones?**

Menopausal or post-menopausal women should consider hormone replacement therapy, with the exception of women in the following situations:

a. women with known or suspected tumours of the type that thrive on estrogen, such as certain breast cancers;
b. women who are pregnant;
c. women with vaginal bleeding of an unknown origin;
d. women with clots in the vein or with a tendency to thrombophlebitis.

As well, women who have gall bladder disease, jaundice, liver disease, a fibroid in the uterus, hypertension, or fibrocystic disease of the breast should, if they undertake hormone replacement therapy, do so with caution.

In almost all other instances, hormone replacement therapy can be considered:

1. to reverse the annoying symptoms of hot flashes;
2. to counteract the development of atrophic vaginitis and urinary symptoms;
3. to counter the inevitable thinning and weakening of bones, called osteoporosis;
4. to reduce the possibility of psychological problems such as depression.

Of course, hormone replacement therapy is not advised for women who don't need it, and is inappropriate for those who consider it unsafe.

If your partner is menopausal or post-menopausal and hormone replacement therapy has not been considered, it should be.

- **Is there any treatment other than replacement hormones for women who suffer hot flashes?**

Bellergal tablets, containing the sedative phenobarbital; ergotamine, a drug that counteracts the sympathetic nervous system; and belladonna, a drug that counteracts the parasympathetic nervous system, have all been tried with some success. Clonidine, a pill used to treat high blood pressure – in a dosage that would be ineffective for hypertension (0.05 mg twice daily) – has reduced the frequency and severity of the flushing attacks. Progesterone (Provera), at a dosage of 20 mg per day, has also been used to treat hot flashes. The results with these preparations are not as consistent as the results obtained with hormone replacement therapy.

- **Why aren't you worried about estrogen in replacement hormones since you worry about estrogen in contraceptive pills?**

Hormone replacement in menopausal women attempts to replace what the body no longer produces. Contraceptive pills attempt to distort normal female hormone levels so that a normal body process (ovulation) does not occur.

The dosages of estrogen in replacement hormones is significantly different from the dosage in contraceptive pills. An appropriate hormonal regime for the menopausal woman is 0.65 mg of the estrogen Premarin for the first twenty-five days of the month, and 5 mg of the progesterone Provera for days sixteen to twenty-five. A woman taking contraceptive pills, on the other hand, would be taking five to twelve times this amount of estrogen each month.

- **Can a man who has had a sex-change operation have a baby?**

It is theoretically possible to implant an embryo inside a man, administer hormones to simulate pregnancy levels, and thus have a male transsexual carry a baby. There has been a case of a woman without a uterus who had a baby; the embryo and its placenta grew on the abdominal wall. But men do not have ovaries, so such a pregnancy would require daily monitoring of hormone levels. Theoretically, a pregnancy is possible, but practically, it is not.

- **Has there never been a successful female-to-male sex change?**

Isolated cases of patients who are pleased with their decisions have been reported. But a result that is cosmetically, functionally, and sexually satisfactory has yet to occur.

- **Christine Jorgensen and René Richards had successful sex-change operations. Don't these success stories justify the procedure?**

If health-care allocations were not an issue, this argument would be convincing. But sex-change operations are extraordinarily expensive. When the costs are paid for by public funds, this operation is not a high priority. Canadian transsexuals are lobbying for more care and are considering court action to make hospitals perform the operation.

9

Sexually Transmitted Diseases

A generation ago, an infectious disease acquired from sexual contact was called a venereal disease. Two of these diseases, syphilis and gonorrhea, became well-known to the public. There was much less familiarity with the other so-called venereal diseases – chancroid, lymphogranuloma venereum, and granuloma inguinale – because they were considered tropical diseases and, therefore, less relevant to people of the Western world.

The old term venereal disease has been replaced by the term sexually transmitted disease, or STD. STDs include a much wider collection of illnesses than did the old category. Included in the group are chlamydia, trichomonas, genital herpes, genital warts, and AIDS (acquired immune deficiency syndrome). There are other illnesses that may or may not be sexually transmitted, such as: yeast infections, bacterial vaginitis, scabies, pubic lice, hepatitis B, and cancer of the cervix. This chapter attempts to clarify all available information on STDs.

Today, men and women have little fear of the traditional venereal diseases because they know that modern medicine can almost always cure them. What people do fear, to the point of paranoia, are genital herpes, because control is uncertain and there is no cure, and AIDS, because it can kill. There is less concern about the other sexually transmitted diseases, although they, too, have disturbing effects.

The Traditional Venereal Diseases

Syphilis

Effective treatment for syphilis has been available only for the last fifty years, but the scourge of syphilis has been around for centuries. The English called it the French Disease; the French, I suspect, called it the English Disease. Every country had it, and no country had a cure for it.

The causative micro-organism can only be identified using a special microscope, by means of a technique called darkfield illumination. The effect is like looking into a dark room in which the bacteria, unique in their large size and spiral shape, appear as dancing lights. This microscopic identification is important, because *Treponema pallidum*, the bacteria that causes syphilis, cannot be grown in the laboratory for purposes of identification.

The syphilis bacteria is transferred from an infected person to an uninfected person through sexual intercourse. Usually, nothing happens for three weeks after exposure, but the incubation period can be as little as ten or as long as sixty days. Then a sore, with distinct features, appears on the genitals where the bacteria has invaded its new host.

This sore, called a chancre, looks like a miniature crater with rough, hard edges. The surface of the crater is pink and oozes a watery discharge. There may be one or several of these sores, and there are painless enlarged lymph nodes nearby in the groin. These nodes are readily palpable to the examining fingers. This primary stage lasts one to five weeks.

After the sore or sores have healed, there may be no obvious evidence of any disease for two to ten weeks. Then a widespread measles-like rash appears and lasts for days, only to disappear completely without treatment. This rash is called the secondary stage. Untreated patients may get attacks of the rash for up to two years.

The disease then enters what is called the latent phase. During the first two years of this period, the patient is infectious, but after two years there is almost no chance of passing on the disease. During this latent period, which can last a lifetime, there may be no further evidence of the disease, or there may be signs of progressive disease in different parts of the body. There can be heart disease, mainly of the heart valves; blood vessel disease, usually a blowout of an artery; damage to the spinal cord at the place where sensations from the legs are carried to the brain; and brain damage that is commonly associated with insanity.

The diagnosis is made by looking for the bacteria in the watery discharge of the primary sore and, indirectly, by checking for the antibodies in the blood that appear about five weeks after the initial exposure. The blood test is known as the VDRL test.

The VDRL (venereal disease research laboratory) test is the most common, but it is not totally accurate. One out of four will test negative in the early stages of the disease. Some people will test positive, not because they have syphilis, but because of malaria, leprosy, lupus, and even after smallpox vaccination.

Syphilis is simply treated with one good dose of penicillin, 2.4 million units intramuscularly. When the patient is allergic to penicillin, tetracycline or erythromycin at a dosage of one 500 mg tablet, four times a day for fifteen days, is prescribed and is equally effective. The effectiveness of the treatment is signalled by changes in the antibodies in the blood. It is not uncommon for antibodies to remain in the blood for three or four years after treatment, although the carrier is not contagious. It is best if the disease is diagnosed and treated in its primary stage, but progression can be halted when the disease is treated even in its secondary or tertiary stage.

Syphilis is re-emerging in the United States, coincident with rising poverty, illegal drugs, and prostitution. Syphilis is also seen more and more in the HIV-positive population.

Gonorrhea

The bacteria that causes gonorrhea may be less damaging to the many different organs of the body than that causing syphilis, but it has an insidious capacity to thrive and multiply in the moist, oxygen-deprived lining of the urethra of men and women. Laboratories that grow the Neisseria gonorrhoeae bacteria must duplicate these conditions. In the old days, labs grew the bacteria on a blood-and-gelatin surface of a culture jar that was depleted of its oxygen by having a lighted candle burn out inside it. If the environment is not moist and oxygen-deprived, the bacteria dies, which is why health-care professionals often laugh when patients suggest that their infection was acquired from a toilet seat or from a swimming pool. More likely, since this bacteria can live in the genital tract of some men and women without causing symptoms, the cause is a silent carrier.

The incubation period for gonorrhea ranges from one day to fourteen days, but can be longer. As a rule, the shorter the incubation period, the more virulent the attack. Half the people infected will have a copious green and yellow discharge

– from the urethra in men and from the vagina in women. Twenty-five per cent will have a more watery discharge, more like that seen in other forms of urethritis. Twenty-five per cent will have no symptoms at all and become silent carriers.

Gonorrhea is diagnosed by identifying gonorrhea bacteria within the white blood cells. The bacteria is known as a Gram negative diplococcus, which means that when a smear on a microscope slide is stained with Gram's stain, the bacteria appears red rather than blue, and appears in pairs. The diagnosis is confirmed by growing bacteria in the laboratory from a swab taken from the urethra or vagina.

Most cases of gonorrhea respond to penicillin (4.8 million units into any muscle along with 1 g of probenecid by mouth). Probenecid prolongs the action of penicillin by blocking its elimination from the kidney. Amoxicillin can be given by mouth 3 g all at once, along with 1 g of probenecid. Amoxicillin is a new form of penicillin, equally effective, and preferred by people who abhor needles. Tetracyline (500 mg by mouth four times a day for two weeks) can be substituted when the patient is allergic to penicillin or amoxicillin. A rare strain of the bacteria produces a chemical that inactivates penicillin. This strain has to be treated with another antibiotic called spectinomycin (2 g intramuscularly).

Recent reports from the United States suggest there are one million new cases of gonorrhea every year, with more than 20 per cent resistant to the usual antibiotics. Ceftriaxone (Rocephin), 125 mg intramuscularly, cefixime (Suprax), 400 mg by mouth, ciprofloxacin (Cipro), 400 mg by mouth, or ofloxacin (Floxin), 400 mg by mouth, along with coincident treatment of possible chlamydia, are becoming the drugs of choice.

A swab from the urethra, 2.5 cm (1 inch) from the opening, should be cultured a week after treatment to ensure that the disease has been successfully eradicated. Gonorrhea can and should be cured in all instances.

Every new case of gonorrhea must be reported to the health authorities, who will trace all the patient's sexual contacts. Only in this way can we eliminate the silent pool of carriers, which is the greatest threat for spreading the disease. The use of condoms can also help contain the spread of gonorrhea.

"Tropical" Venereal Diseases

The tropical venereal diseases discussed below are exceptionally rare in the Western world. The three cases I have seen in over thirty-two years of practice have been carried by visitors from tropical countries.

For anyone unfortunate enough to acquire one of these illnesses, it is encouraging to remember that all are responsive to commonly used antibacterial agents.

Chancroid

This disease is caused by a bacteria called *Hemophilus ducreyi*. The incubation period of chancroid ranges from three to ten days. A low-grade fever and malaise may then occur, followed by an ulcer (like that seen in syphilis except the edges are soft) and enlarged and painful lymph nodes in the groin (unlike those seen in syphilis). The disease responds to sulfonamide (Trimethoprim-sulfamethoxazole double-strength tablet twice a day for ten days). Tetracycline or erythromycin can be substituted for the sulfonamide when there is intolerance or allergy to the sulfa.

The recommended treatment for chancroid is azithromycin (Zithromax), 1 g by mouth as a single dose, or ceftriaxone (Rocephin), 250 mg intramuscularly as a single dose, or erythromycin (Eryc), 500 mg by mouth four times a day for seven days.

Lymphogranuloma Venereum

This venereal disease is caused by a particular strain of the chlamydia bacteria. The incubation period ranges from three to fourteen days. The most characteristic feature of this disease is that the lymph nodes in the groin enlarge to such an extent that they mat together, invade the overlying skin, turning it purple, and then break through to the outside. The disease can be treated with sulfonamides, tetracycline, or erythromycin, but the recommended regime at present is doxycycline (Vibramycin), 100 mg twice a day by mouth for twenty-one days.

Granuloma Inguinale

This disease has features of the two diseases described above – large matted nodes in the groin and soft-edged ulcers. It is caused by another family of bacteria, called *C. granulomatis*. The disease has an incubation period ranging from eight to eighty days, and it responds to the standard antibiotic treatment previously described.

Today's Common STDs

Chlamydia Urethritis

Chlamydia urethritis was, until recently, difficult to diagnose because the laboratory technique used to culture bacteria cannot be used. The chlamydia organism has been identified as a tiny bacteria that can live only inside a live cell. Until this was discovered, clear urethral discharge not attributable to gonorrhea was called non-specific urethritis, an inflammation of the urethra associated with discharge. Now it is known that the chlamydia bacteria is responsible for most cases of non-specific urethritis and, also, for most cases of epididymitis, a painful swelling of the epididymis. In women, chlamydia infection is a major cause of spontaneous abortion, tubal pregnancy, pelvic inflammatory disease, and infertility.

But 50 per cent of all cases of chlamydial infections are totally free of any symptoms. In a study of eight hundred women who had come for their annual pap smear at a government health centre in Montreal, 7.5 per cent had chlamydia without knowing it. The infection was seen twice as often in women who were under twenty-five years of age and had a red cervix or inflammation. Thus, it might be prudent for men and women who are sexually promiscuous to have themselves tested for the chlamydial organism.

The 50 per cent who develop symptoms do so after an incubation period of one to three weeks. These men and women experience a burning sensation while urinating and develop a discharge that is sticky and either clear or creamy.

Chlamydial infection has become pervasive in Western society. The real incidence is unknown, but more than 5 per cent of all pregnant women are affected, and chlamydia is the most common cause of eye infection in the newborn.

Recently, detection kits have become commercially available. The test detects chlamydial protein by binding it to a prepared antibody that is linked to an enzyme. When the antibody is taken up, the enzyme changes colour. This test does not work as well when the infection is mild. Tests done on urine were not sufficiently accurate until recently, but the latest report suggests accurate diagnosis with a urine sample.

Treatment of chlamydial infection is simple enough, though. The disease responds to tetracyline, 500 mg four times a day for ten to fourteen days. Other medications that can be used as well include erythromycin, second-generation tetracyclines such as doxycycline (Vibramycin) or minocycline (Minocin), and the sulfonamides such as the sulfamethoxazole/trimethoprim combination (Septra or Bactrim). Seven days' treatment with ofloxacin seems equally effective, but the recommended regime in 1995 is doxycycline (Vibramycin), 100 mg by mouth twice a day for seven days, or a single 1 g dose of azithromycin (Zithromax) by mouth.

Ureaplasma

Ureaplasma is an unusual and confusing bacteria. Unlike most bacteria, it has no cell wall, but, unlike a virus, it is sensitive to antibiotics. In recent years microbiologists have developed a specific test for ureaplasma. The question is: If you have it, do you treat it?

Seventy per cent of people with ureaplasma have no problems. Some have symptoms which come and go over the years. There have been cases of spontaneous abortion, infection of the Fallopian tubes, and infection of the epididymis when the only possible pathogen that tested positive was ureaplasma.

Doctors researching the field treat ureaplasma only when three conditions pertain: when they can see signs of infection; when the patient reports symptoms; and when all the other tests for STDs are negative and only the ureaplasma test is positive.

Signs of infection in women are a red cervix and a puslike discharge from the cervix. Symptoms in women are a transparent vaginal discharge (which may vary from a lot to a little), a burning sensation when urinating, and discomfort during intercourse, because the vaginal skin becomes delicate and fragile due to the discharge. In men, there may be a clear discharge from the penis.

The treatment used today is tetracycline. Based on a culture after a course of treatment, 75 to 85 per cent of the patients are cured. Oddly, though, patients often continue to report the same symptoms. Tetracyclines frequently cause stomach upset. Lab data suggests that a new family of antibiotics, called quinolones, are a promising agent for ureaplasma. Although there are as yet no clinical studies on the use of quinolones for ureaplasma, studies on the use of quinolones for chlamydia, a similar bacteria, show a cure rate of 70 per cent. Some people are free of symptoms after a while with no treatment at all. Sometimes the symptoms reoccur, and sometimes they do not. Ureaplasma is considered a grey area of medicine.

Trichomoniasis

The organism *Trichomonas vaginalis* is a common cause of a frothy, itchy, malodorous, whitish green vaginal discharge in women. It looks like a teardrop-shaped miniature water insect, with a flat body and a tail that causes it to wiggle under the microscope. It can live in the male genital tract in the urethra or prostate, but often causes no symptoms in men. Trichomoniasis, the disease caused by this organism, can ping-pong between sexual partners, and is thus considered sexual in origin. I have difficulty accepting a sexual cause in all cases, however, since I have seen the problem in sexually abstinent women and, furthermore, it is a disproportionately female complaint. No reasonable explanation for this sex distribution has been offered. Recently it has been reported that these unicellular organisms can survive for up to one day in chlorinated water, hot tubs, and weak soap solutions, thus raising the possibility of non-sexual transmission.

The diagnosis is made by recognizing the protozoa under a microscope. Treatment consists of a drug called metronidazole

(Flagyl), 2 g by mouth as a single dose or 500 mg by mouth twice a day for seven days. If the woman has a regular sexual partner, they must both undergo treatment. Flagyl is known to cause cancer in rats, but is not considered harmful in humans. I feel that the drug presents a very slight risk, but I recommend it to patients with trichomoniasis since it is the only drug we know that will clear it up. The drug, however, is considered too dangerous for women to take during early pregnancy, because the risk of malformed babies is greater.

The malodorous vaginal discharge associated with trichomoniasis can be confused with the discharge of vaginosis, due to anaerobic or non-oxygen-requiring bacteria, and vaginitis due to yeast infection, like candida.

The pH (acidity) of the discharge will be higher than 4.5 when the discharge is due to anaerobic bacteria. When the discharge on a slide is diluted with a drop of 10 per cent potassium hydroxide (KOH), a fishy odour should suggest trichomoniasis or bacterial vaginosis. The typical branched appearance of yeast will be readily seen with potassium hydroxide.

Venereal Warts

The scientific name for a venereal wart is *condylomata acuminata*. As in all other warts, the cause is a virus that, as might be suspected, can easily be passed from one person to another by intimate sexual relations.

The wart looks like a tiny pink cauliflower and is easily recognized in men. It is much more difficult to see in women, because the wart is similar in colour to the vaginal wall and because the corrugations of the vagina camouflage the wart. The warts can be identified more readily when painted with vinegar, which makes them whiter, and by using a magnifying glass. In men, the warts can be located on the head of the penis, on the shaft of the penis, on the scrotum, around the anus, at the opening of the urethra, and even inside the urethra. In women, the warts can be near the clitoris, on the outer or inner lips, around the anus, at the opening of the vagina and even deep inside it, and on the cervix. There can be tremendous variation in their size, ranging from a few millimetres to a few centimetres across. If there has been mouth-to-genital contact, there can be warts inside the mouth in either sex.

Venereal warts can be treated in a number of ways. A chemical called podophyllin can be applied directly to the wart. Commonly, a 20 per cent solution of the drug, mixed with tincture of benzoin to make it sticky, is dabbed on the wart and the centimetre (approx. 0.5 inches) of skin surrounding it. After one to four hours, it is then washed off. The podophyllin treatment can be acutely painful when applied to delicate tissue such as the urinary opening or head of the penis. Recently the active ingredient in podophyllin, called podofilox (Condyline), has become available. It may be less irritating to the surrounding skin. A 0.5 per cent solution is applied with a Q-tip twice daily for three days, and the treatment is repeated four days later. As many as four cycles of treatment can be tried.

The warts can be burned off with an application of frozen nitrogen, by electro-cautery, or with a laser. The frozen nitrogen method burns an area larger than necessary, and electro-cautery requires some form of anaesthetic. The laser treatment will eventually become the treatment of choice, as it is totally painless, but most hospitals are not yet equipped for it. Improperly applied laser treatment can cause horrendous complications, however, as in one man who required skin grafting to cover the burned area and remains impotent from damage to the nerve. But accidents like this are most uncommon.

When the warts are inside the male urethra, overly aggressive treatment such as that done with electrocautery can cause a stricture of the passage. Weekly instillations of the anti-cancer drugs 5-fluoro-uracil or thio-tepa, instead, have successfully eradicated the warts after about five treatments. When the wart is on a woman's cervix, it is often wise to perform a biopsy, as venereal warts have been linked to the development of cervical cancer.

Even when there is no longer any visible evidence of venereal warts, they can reoccur without re-exposure. And when left neglected for a long time, giant warts measured in inches may cover the genitalia. These are associated with cancer formation at the site.

I remember using electrocautery and general anaesthetic to burn off innumerable venereal warts around the genitalia and anus of one patient. Then, remembering that there was another one inside his mouth, I moved to the head of the table and applied the instrument to the wart located there. The nurse, watching me, was alarmed. "You just used that instrument on the guy's ass," she exclaimed. "I know," I replied. "It's all right, electrocautery is self-sterilizing." She gave me a look of utter disgust. I don't know if it was my technique that did it or the nature of this particular health problem.

I advise my patients to check themselves for the warts for as long as one year after successful eradication. As the incubation period for condyloma can be as long as six months, I consider them cured only after one whole year of freedom from new warts.

Genital Herpes

Genital herpes is the third most-common sexually transmitted disease today. Gonorrhea is still number one, and chlamydia is number two.

The causative organism is a herpes simplex virus that exists in two forms, called type 1 and type 2, with only a minor chemical difference between them. The type 1 virus is associated 90 per cent of the time with blisters around the mouth and 10 per cent of the time with blisters on the genitals. The type 2 virus is associated 90 per cent of the time with genital blisters, and 10 per cent of the time with blisters on the mouth.

After the initial direct transference of the herpes virus from an infected person onto the skin or genital lining of an uninfected person (lesion to hand to genital, or lesion to mouth to genital), there is a two- to ten-day incubation period. During this time there may be pain and a pins-and-needles feeling at the site of the viral transfer. Then flu-like symptoms develop – fever, headaches, muscle aches, and swollen lymph nodes. Later, at the site of transfer, tiny blisters appear on a reddened base. In women, the blisters occur on the vulva, vagina, and cervix. In men the common sites are the head of the penis, foreskin, and shaft of the penis. After a week or two, the blisters burst and become tiny painful erosions or ulcers. A dry crust forms over the ulcers about twenty days later. Between the time the blisters break and the time they crust over, the virus is contagious and can be transmitted to others.

It takes about three weeks for herpes ulcers to heal. After this time, the painful, enlarged lymph nodes that have developed in the groin also subside and the attack is over.

But even when there is no further evidence of an attack, the virus remains in the body, inside the nerve cells. Attacks recur in 80 per cent of patients, but they are usually milder than the first episode.

The diagnosis is made by simple inspection. If there is any doubt, the diagnosis can be double-checked by scraping material from the base of the blister, staining it, and examining it under a microscope. If it is a case of herpes, the scraping will contain giant cells with many nuclei. These giant cells are also seen in chicken pox scrapings and in shingles, but there is little confusion with these illnesses when the overall picture is considered. The diagnosis can also be confirmed by viral tissue culture.

There is no curative treatment for genital herpes. A drug called acyclovir (Zovirax) was introduced in 1985. It does not kill the virus but slows its rate of reproduction. Acyclovir cream applied to the blisters decreases pain and shortens the duration of the attack. It is considered effective for the first attack but of questionable value for subsequent attacks. Acyclovir pills have also hit the market. A 200 mg tablet taken five times a day for seven to ten days lessens the severity of the attack and speeds up healing. Frequent recurrent attacks may also be lessened by taking the pills five times a day for five days, then two pills three times a day for five days, then four pills twice a day for five days, then one pill twice a day for up to six months. In the short time Acyclovir has been available, there has been no report of any dangerous side effects, but the medication is expensive.

A young lady once asked me whether I approved of her starting a relationship with a man who had a history of genital herpes. I told her that when blisters were present, abstinence or the use of condoms could not guarantee safety if there was still intimate sexual contact. I figured, though, that when there is a caring relationship, it transcends an illness like herpes, which is never fatal.

AIDS (Acquired Immune Deficiency Syndrome)

The first ever case of AIDS was reported in America in 1981. Since then, AIDS has become the most serious epidemic of the last fifty years.

Information on AIDS is continually changing, and it is difficult to have perspective in the middle of an epidemic. More than ninety-five countries of the world are affected by the disease, and several million people have already died of AIDS. According to the World Health Organization (WHO), forty million people could become HIV-positive by the year 2000, up from some ten million today. In the first edition of this book (published in 1988), I stated that a hundred thousand cases of AIDS had been reported since the discovery of the virus in 1981, and five to ten million people were carriers of the virus. The next hundred thousand cases were reported in the following two years.

The numbers are expected to rise more slowly in the United States, from one million HIV-positive today to one and a half million at the end of the century. It has already become the most frequent cause of death in New York City for women between twenty and twenty-five and men between twenty-five and forty. As in the United States, the disease in Canada is appearing more and more in the heterosexual population. The WHO expects the rate of new infection to increase at a far higher rate from heterosexual activity than from homosexual activity, and more women than men will be affected.

The control of this epidemic will depend on the development of a vaccine or a drastic change in sexual habits. The Surgeon General of the United States has estimated that it will take another thirty years to develop an effective vaccine. This is because the AIDS virus mutates and, like the flu virus, each new strain requires a separate vaccine. Since it took twenty years to develop a vaccine against hepatitis B, it is expected that a vaccine for this even more complicated virus will take longer.

It is difficult to know whether the general population is frightened enough of the AIDS epidemic to modify its sexual behaviour, but partner screening and the use of condoms appear imperative to control the epidemic.

Recovering the virus from infected tissue and growing it in tissue culture may seem the most logical way to study this disease. Theoretically it is possible, but it is not done, since the culture technique is difficult, expensive, and generally unavailable. But the spin-off from the massive research effort to discover a cure for AIDS will likely advance our understanding of other disease processes such as cancer and transplantation rejection. A breakthrough in cancer control might well become the serendipitous bonus of this modern-day scourge.

The causative virus has now been isolated and characterized. This virus, originally designated as HTLV-III (human T-lymphotropic virus-III) in the United States, and LAV (lymphadenopathy-associated virus) in France, is now known internationally as HIV (for human immunodeficiency virus). The HIV virus attacks a particular family of blood cells, called T-helper lymphocytes, which are indispensable in producing certain immune responses. If all the T-helper lymphocytes are destroyed, the body cannot resist certain serious lung infections or fight against the cancerous process, and full-blown AIDS ensues.

Right now, there is no simple test that tells whether or not a person has AIDS. What is tested, instead, is whether a person has been exposed to the AIDS virus (HIV) and has developed antibodies. The ELISA test (enzyme-linked immunosorbent assay) is the blood test used to determine the presence of antibodies. When the AIDS virus is present, the antibody is bound, and this reaction changes the colour of the enzyme linked to the antibody. Ninety-five per cent of people who have had a sexual or blood contact with the AIDS virus produce detectable levels of the antibody, making them HIV positive. Five per cent do not produce antibodies, even though they have the AIDS virus.

Historically, the people with the most risk of contracting AIDS were homosexuals, intravenous drug users who shared needles, Haitians, and haemophiliacs and other blood-product recipients. This has changed to some extent in that blood transfusions are now safer. All donations at blood-donor clinics are screened for AIDS antibodies with the ELISA test, and blood that tests positive is not used. Unfortunately, the test does not identify exposed donors who have not yet developed antibodies, nor does it screen out the 5 per cent who have the virus without antibodies. Nevertheless, since the Red Cross began testing donors, there have been virtually no cases of transmission due to transfusion.

The AIDS virus is transmitted through blood, semen, and cervical-vaginal secretions. It has also been found in urine, breast milk, tears, and saliva, but there has not yet been a documented case of transmission from these sources. The virus has been transmitted from infected mother to child during, or shortly after, birth. It used to be thought that the AIDS virus was transmitted only through anal intercourse. Now it is known to be transmitted through vaginal intercourse as well. No case of transmission through oral intercourse has yet been confirmed. Researchers have shown, however, that the AIDS virus behaves like the hepatitis B virus. And, since hepatitis B has been transmitted by oral sex alone, from man to man or man to woman, it is presumed that the AIDS virus can be transmitted in the same way.

The AIDS virus is known to have been transmitted in a single encounter and is thought to be an easily transmitted virus. The odds of infection from a single encounter are not known.

Condoms are suggested as a barrier to transmission. The

Journal of the American Medical Association published a laboratory study showing that the AIDS virus cannot pass through
either a synthetic or natural-skin condom. A University of
Miami clinical study also showed the protective value of
condoms. When condoms were used, only one out of ten of
the partners of AIDS patients developed antibodies. This is a
striking contrast to the twelve out of fourteen partners who
developed antibodies when condoms were not used. These
condom studies suggest that continued sexual contact without
preventative measures will result in AIDS transmission, and
that sexual contact with barrier contraceptives is, short of
abstinence, the safest means of protection known.

Thus, the only safe sex is with a partner never exposed to
the AIDS virus. When a person has had sex with other partners, there is always a theoretical chance of previous exposure, even with a negative HIV blood test, and condoms
provide the best protection. Unprotected sex or the sharing of
needles are unacceptable practices today.

There have been reports in the popular magazines that the
spermicide Nonoxynol-9 inactivates the AIDS virus, but there
are no scientific studies to support this claim. In laboratory
studies, the AIDS virus has been killed by detergents, soaps,
alcohol, and sterilization. The most effective disinfectant in
the studies is a 0.5 per cent solution of hypochlorite, the
chemical in laundry bleach.

Perhaps one of the most frightening aspects of AIDS is the
possibility of silent transmission. A person can be incubating
the virus, not have sufficient antibodies to test positive, and
still transmit the disease.

Of the first hundred thousand cases of AIDS in the United
States, 4 per cent were due to heterosexual contact; in the
next hundred thousand, this had risen to 6 per cent. Although
heterosexual transmission is increasing, the vast majority of

people getting AIDS right now are gay men and drug users who share needles.

On the positive side, scientists who have studied people living with AIDS patients have shown that, apart from actual intimate sexual contact, transmission does not occur. In the families studied, the virus has not been transmitted by hugging, kissing, or by sharing kitchen and bathroom facilities.

Progress of the Disease

People who have had contact with the AIDS virus will develop antibodies, or seroconvert, one week to six months later. This means that after a suspected contact, a person can have the ELISA antibody test to check if he or she is infected. If the test is positive, the person has been exposed; if negative, the person is probably not infected, although they can seroconvert any time up to six months after exposure to the virus.

If a person tests positive on the ELISA test, it is repeated and reconfirmed in another test, called the Western Blot. This test looks for a different protein in the AIDS virus. Even if both tests are positive, the person will not necessarily get AIDS; the tests do not confirm that the person is infectious or infected, only that the person has been exposed to the AIDS virus. The only hard data we have on the percentage of people with anti-bodies who actually get AIDS is based on a three-year study of homosexual men in New York City. Of these seropositive men, 34.2 per cent developed AIDS. AIDS experts feel that many more of these subjects likely developed AIDS after the end of the three-year period. The current estimate is that 30 to 70 per cent of those who are seropositive will develop AIDS.

A person may have the AIDS virus for many years without feeling sick. A recent English study (1994) of 111 haemophil-iac patients reported that 25 per cent of men who seroconvert can expect to live twenty to twenty-five years after testing positive. A similar study in California suggested that 15 per cent of the HIV-positive population would live up to another twenty years. People are counselled on the presumption that testing positive for antibodies means they may transmit the disease.

When the AIDS symptoms appear, they may do so in a variety of ways. Most often, the seropositive patient will develop what is called the AIDS Related Complex (ARC) before developing full-blown AIDS. ARC is defined by a collection of symptoms and lab findings. The symptoms are a three-month history of any two of the following:

1. fever in excess of 38°C (100.4°F),
2. night sweats,
3. ten-pound weight loss (or 10 per cent of body weight),
4. diarrhoea,
5. fatigue,
6. enlarged lymph nodes in more than two areas other than the groin.

The lab findings can include:

1. decreased red blood cells, decreased white blood count, decreased platelets (tiny blood-cell products necessary for normal clotting),
2. increased immune responses such as gamma globulin, which is the protein base for all antibodies that fight disease,
3. failure to respond to the tuberculosis skin test and other skin tests.

Often, the clinical manifestations are yeast infections, unexplained mouth infections, or shingles, which show as painful, pigmented blisters following the distribution of the nerve. Some people who develop this complex may die from it. Others will go on to develop full-blown AIDS, which is always fatal.

Some patients get AIDS without any preliminary stages. They get a specific form of pneumonia (*Pneumocystis carinii*), or a specific form of skin cancer (Kaposi's sarcoma). The pneumonia in AIDS is like any other pneumonia except that the patient seldom improves. The cancer in AIDS also behaves no differently.

A small percentage of seropositive patients get neurological symptoms when they get AIDS. Some patients manifest only neurological symptoms – a progressive loss of cerebral function accompanied by motor and behavioural disturbances. In a study of patients with only neurological symptoms, half developed full-scale AIDS and half died without exhibiting any other signs of AIDS.

AIDS is invariably fatal, but it is not clear how many HIV-positive people develop AIDS; many educated guesses in the past have proven wrong. When there has been exposure to the AIDS virus, medications like zidovudine (AZT or Retrovir) may delay becoming HIV positive, delay development of symptoms, reduce symptoms, and prolong life. Other drugs like AZT are about to be launched or are being developed.

These positive trends, undramatic as they may appear, should change the laws regarding HIV testing. A patient's right to decide whether to be tested for the virus or not made sense when no therapy was available. But maintaining this stance today is unfair to health-care workers who may choose prophylactic treatment after an accidental exposure.

Other Possible STDs

There are a number of other diseases that may be considered sexually transmitted because of the manner in which they are spread.

Hepatitis

Hepatitis B does not affect sexual organs, but it spreads much like AIDS, and the resulting severe damage to the liver can be fatal. Hepatitis B can certainly be acquired non-sexually, by a contaminated needle or contaminated blood, but the virus can also be transmitted sexually. Hepatitis B vaccine is available and should be taken by the sexual partners of people who have, or are carriers of, the virus. The vaccine is made from the plasma of patients with the hepatitis B virus. These patients are often gay, so people are often fearful that they may pick up the AIDS virus when they get the vaccine. This is not possible, but this concern is only one of many misconceptions about hepatitis B.

Until ten years ago, doctors recognized only two kinds of viral hepatitis. One was called infectious hepatitis, which is now called hepatitis A, and the other was called serum hepatitis, which is now called hepatitis B. Two more viral agents are now known, one called non-A, non-B, and the other called hepatitis D virus, an incomplete virus that causes disease only when hepatitis B virus is also present.

Hepatitis A

The hepatitis A virus is acquired by eating or drinking food, water, milk, or shellfish contaminated by faeces containing the virus. (The virus inside shellfish may not be destroyed by cooking when the shell is intact and does not open.) There is an incubation period of four weeks, after which low-grade fever, tiredness, loss of appetite, nausea, vomiting, headaches, and muscle aches appear. Within a week, the urine turns dark, the stool turns light, pain and discomfort develop in the upper right side of the abdomen, where the liver is located, and the skin and the whites of the eyes turn yellow. After several weeks, most patients slowly recover and develop a lifetime immunity to further attacks.

Hepatitis B

Five per cent of the world's population, or two hundred million people, are chronically infected with the hepatitis B virus. The virus has been found in the body secretions of these people: the saliva, tears, sweat, semen, vaginal secretions, breast milk, urine, and faeces. Most transmission is by contaminated needles, sexual intimacy, or into the newborn through a contaminated birth canal.

Once the virus is acquired, the incubation period can vary from one to three months, and, rarely, up to six months. The incubation period is shorter when the virus is inoculated into a cut or a needle prick, and longer when the transmission is sexual or oral.

Hepatitis B infection can then take an acute or a chronic course. In the acute course, the clinical disease is like that of hepatitis A, and recovery occurs after about two to three months. Five to ten per cent of patients with the acute course will remain chronically infected with the virus. In the chronic course, the beginnings of the disease are blurred, and the malaise persists for a long time. Eventually the liver may shrivel up, a condition called cirrhosis, or it may develop a cancer.

Hepatitis B can be prevented by a newly developed vaccine. The vaccine was developed from the plasma of hepatitis B carriers, who have a non-infectious viral coat protein in their plasma. The plasma is boiled, chemically treated to remove other proteins, and mixed with formalin. These processes eliminate any possibility of contamination with the live AIDS virus, but do not affect the function of the hepatitis B vaccine.

Protection from hepatitis B is due to the vaccinated person's ability to produce protective antibodies. When there is an accidental exposure to the hepatitis B virus, such as a mishap in the operating room, or a sexual exposure, and there may not be sufficient time to stimulate the patient to make antibodies by vaccinating him, hyperimmune serum or serum from patients that have already produced the antibodies is used. Such a treatment can abort an attack. A person in a debilitated state may not be able to produce the antibodies.

Scabies and Lice

Scabies, known for its tremendous itchiness, is caused by a tiny "insect" that burrows just under the skin. Scabies can be spread from one person to another by sexual relations. Lindane lotion or cream, popularly known as Kwellada, applied regularly over a period of ten to twelve hours, is usually curative.

Pubic lice, or crabs, also known for their itchiness, are mites that survive on pubic hair. Close contact can spread the lice from one person to another. Lindane can be used, but skin application of a drug called piperonyl butoxide may be less irritating and equally effective.

Jock Itch

The upper inner thigh and surrounding area of the groin is prone to the fungus known as ringworm (*Tinea cruris*) and yeast (Candida) infections. This causes an itchy irritation of the skin, known as jock itch. If an anti-fungal or anti-yeast treatment is not applied, there can be further erosion of the skin from scratching, resulting in secondary bacterial infection. Both fungus and yeast infections can be spread from one area of the body to another, but neither organism is very contagious, and transmission, even by sexual contact, is rare.

Yeast Infection

In women, yeast infection of the vulva and vagina is not uncommon. This can occur with or without sexual contact, in women taking an oral antibiotic, in diabetics, women on the pill, and women who do not routinely wear cotton underwear. There is often an intense vaginal itch and a discharge that is thick, white, and cheesy. This yeast infection can be passed on to the male partner, whose only symptom may be an increased redness in the head and shaft of the penis. An anti-fungal cream such as miconazole (Monistat 7), clotrimazole (Canesten), or nystatin (Mycostatin or Nilstat) is curative.

The anti-fungal preparations currently recommended are miconazole (Monistat 7) 2 per cent cream, intravaginally for seven days; miconazole 200 mg vaginal suppository daily for three days; miconazole 100 mg vaginal suppository daily for seven days; clotrimazole (Canesten) 1 per cent cream intravaginally for seven to fourteen days; clotrimazole 100 mg vaginal tablet for seven days, or 100 mg vaginal tablet twice for three days, or 500 mg vaginal tablet as a single application.

Another common cause of vaginal discharge is infection caused by the *Gardnerella vaginalis* bacteria. A telltale fishy odour after intercourse is a sign of this infection. It is not certain whether it can be transmitted to men. The recommended regimens for bacterial vaginosis are metronidazole (Flagyl) 500 mg orally twice a day for seven days; metronidazole 2 g as a single dose; clindamycin (Dalacin) 2 per cent cream for seven days; metronidazole 0.75 per cent gel intra-vaginally twice a day for five days; clindamycin 300 mg twice a day for seven days.

Finally, a case can be made to suggest that carcinoma of the cervix may be sexual in origin. It has been determined that not one case of cancer of the cervix appeared in ten thousand nuns who were sexually abstinent. There is, on the other hand, statistical evidence that the cancer occurs more frequently in women who have had multiple sex partners. However, a causative factor, presumably associated with the penis, has not been identified, although the human papilloma virus is most suspect.

Questions and Answers

- **Can I get herpes from a person with no obvious sores?**

The risk of transmission is certainly reduced when there are no visible signs, but not totally eliminated. One to fifteen per cent of people with type 2 herpes will transmit the virus without themselves having any visible signs. You can, therefore, be unknowingly infected by your sexual partners.

- **What is the difference between type 1 and type 2 herpes viruses?**

There is a very slight protein difference, detectable in refined laboratory tests. The striking difference is seen in the health problems which result: type 1 virus usually causes fever blisters of the lips; type 2 virus causes genital ulcers.

- **Will tetracycline cure me of chlamydia?**

Yes. It works now, but it may not tomorrow. It used to be that every case of gonorrhea was cured by penicillin. Now there are penicillin-resistant strains of gonorrhea, especially in Southeast Asia.

- **Should I take tetracycline instead of penicillin for gonorrhea?**

Treatment with tetracyline would likely eliminate chlamydia infection which might have been acquired at the same time. But there are gonorrhea infections that resist both penicillin and tetracycline.

- **Could I have got venereal warts from something other than sexual contact?**

It's not likely. Stated another way, it has been shown that 60 per cent of the partners of patients with condyloma develop a venereal wart within a three-month period. The incubation period for this virus ranges from one to six months.

- **I guess I don't have to worry about getting syphilis since it's been eradicated.**

This is simply not so. In certain areas of the world, such as Western Europe and America, more new cases of syphilis are being diagnosed now than a generation ago.

- **Can I avoid STDs by scrubbing with soap and water after sexual relations?**

No! The simplest reliable protection is to use a condom.

- **Haven't French scientists developed an effective treatment for AIDS, and isn't there a new drug that is supposed to be effective?**

French scientists' preliminary results suggested that the immunosuppressive drug Cyclosporin A might help patients with AIDS. Subsequent follow-up of the patients has discounted the early results.

AZT and similar preparations being developed or under preliminary trials may retard the progress of AIDS, but there is still no cure for this disease.

- **Can I sue somebody for knowingly transmitting a STD?**

There are several cases of this nature before the courts. The decisions of the lower courts will, undoubtedly, be appealed, and the final outcome will take years. I suspect that people who knowingly transmit STDs will be prosecuted. But asymptomatic carriers can spread the disease, and the question of their responsibility is a complicated one. Carriers of gonorrhea, herpes, and chlamydia can be asymptomatic, and these are the three most common STDs.

- **Is AIDS more contagious than hepatitis B?**

The hepatitis B virus is much more contagious, but AIDS is deadly.

10

Women

Whatever the impulse – be it evolutionary, sociological, or simply sexual – men and women often come in pairs. It is not surprising, then, that women's private parts affect the rhythm and cycle of men's lives. Yet most men regard women with a degree of uncertainty. Like Professor Higgins in *My Fair Lady*, they wonder, "Why can't a woman be more like a man?" But women are anatomically and hormonally different from men. If you are going to love them, it's a good idea, at the very least, to know how their bodies work.

The Design Question

Women are more susceptible than men to urinary infections because of the design of their urethra. If women could empty their bladders through the belly button, as might have been the design early on in our evolution, it would dramatically reduce female urinary infections. But the original tube from the bladder to the belly button (which is called the urachus, and which is present in-utero) has disappeared, to be replaced by a urethra which drains the bladder from below. Women now have a urethral opening just above the vagina.

A woman's urethral tube is as sensitive and as delicate as the lining of the nose. It runs alongside the vagina, which is as strong as leather and as pliable as a rubber band. Its opening is only inches away from the anus. Because it is easy for bacteria to travel, the proximity of the urethral opening to the vagina and the anus creates sex-associated bladder infections. Bacteria travel from the vagina or the anus to the urethra. Foreplay and thrusting during intercourse often milk the bacteria that are in the urethra into the bladder, where urine provides a good medium for bacterial growth. Bacteria make up 50 per cent of the dry weight of stool, and these bacteria are the most common cause of urinary infection.

Consequently, men should be careful not to put faecal bacteria into the urethra. During foreplay, different fingers should be used when touching the urethra and the anus. During

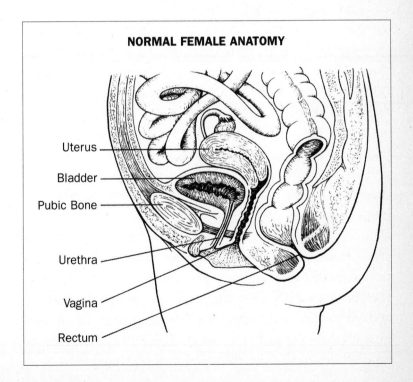

NORMAL FEMALE ANATOMY

Uterus

Bladder

Pubic Bone

Urethra

Vagina

Rectum

cunnilingus the tongue should stop before the anus. Harsh manipulation of the area around the urethral opening can cause painful trauma. In general, remember that the urethra is a delicate structure, and that faecal bacteria, although microscopic, can cause painful urinary infection.

Male consideration during intercourse will reduce female urinary infection but not eliminate it. In women prone to bladder infections, bowel bacteria actually live on the vulva adjacent to the urinary opening. Women less prone to bladder infection seem to have a protective mechanism that prevents bowel bacteria from colonizing this area. In any case, about a quarter of all women between the ages of twenty and forty will have at least one episode of the bladder infection called cystitis, and, of these, 80 per cent will have more than one episode.

"Honeymoon" Cystitis

In most cases of "honeymoon" cystitis, intercourse is the direct cause. Why some women are more vulnerable than others to this problem is not clear. It is not simply a matter of hygiene, although a habit such as wiping forward with toilet paper, instead of wiping backward from the vagina to the anus, could be a contributing factor. It is simply, as I have said, that some women have better defence mechanisms than others, and their immune systems destroy the bacteria that persist in others.

In diagnosing cystitis it is important to know what kind of bowel bacteria is responsible in order to know what medication to use. This is ascertained by a midstream urine culture. Hospital bacteria are very hardy and resist the usual antibiotics. They must be treated by powerful antibiotics administered directly into the bloodstream, or by injections into a muscle, depending on the results of elaborate laboratory testing. Urinary infection acquired in the community, on the other hand, can be eradicated by most anti-bacterial pills, and laboratory testing, although helpful, is not essential. The traditional ten- to fourteen-day treatment is being replaced by a shorter drug regime of three to five days, and even a one-shot six-pill dose is being tried with good results, using drugs such as the trimethoprim-sulfamethoxazole combination or the penicillin type Amoxicillin. A shorter regime assures that the complete dosage will be taken, since a major problem with the traditional treatment has been that women stop taking the drug the moment they feel better.

The traditional treatment offered women with cystitis was a course of antibiotics and instructions to empty the bladder immediately after intercourse, like flushing a toilet after use. Infections continued to recur with this regime, and recently we have learned why. Bacteria that cause cystitis adhere to the wall of the bladder, and flushing is not sufficient to eliminate them. I instruct my patients to swab an antiseptic, such as proviodine, on the vulva daily, to suppress the normal bacterial flora. In addition I prescribe an antibiotic pill, such as nitrofurantoin (50 mg), to be taken a half-hour before intercourse. It may be taken, instead, after intercourse, although that is not as effective. I am impressed by how effective this simple regime has been.

One woman whom I counselled as indicated replied:

"You mean I must take the pill every time I make love?"

"Yes."

"Seven times a day?"

"You're joking."

"I'm not. This is a relationship that just started, and it's going great."

(I still think she was pulling my leg.)

Nitrofurantoin is the drug I favour to treat cystitis, but

almost any antibiotic or antibacterial preparation can be substituted. I choose nitrofurantoin because it specifically targets the urinary tract and is less likely to cause side effects or to develop bacteria resistant to the drug.

Urinary Infections – Pregnancy, Post-Menopause

Silent, or asymptomatic, urinary-tract infections occur in 6 per cent of all pregnant women. Untreated, 40 per cent of these women will develop symptoms and clinical infections of the kidney, whereas none of the treated women develop symptoms of illness. It is a good idea to culture the urine of pregnant women on a regular basis, perhaps once a month.

Urethral problems and bladder infections are common in post-menopausal women. The lower estrogen level causes the walls of the vagina and urethra to be drier and thinner. Injury and irritation from intercourse become more likely as a consequence. Men whose partners have dry and easily irritated vaginas may help solve the problem with water-soluble lubricants such as Lubafax or K-Gel. Water-insoluble lubricants such as Vaseline or mineral oil can cause a reaction and should not be used.

If the urethra gets irritated it may scar, and the scars may interfere with normal evacuation. A bladder partially blocked by a scarred urethra won't be able to empty completely, and will be more prone to infection.

When the bladder becomes infected because of urethral scarring, it is helped by periodic dilatations of the urethra and long-term, low-dose antibacterial treatment, such as nitrofurantoin, 50 mg daily, for several months. If your partner is subject to this problem, she should be offered replacement hormone therapy, using both estrogen and progesterone preparations as discussed in the section on menopause. As it is usually gynecologists who prescribe the hormones and urologists who dilate the urethra and prescribe the antibiotics, the complete treatment, requiring both antibiotics and hormones, is frequently mismanaged.

Often, because the gynecologist sees no gynecological necessity, my patients have not been given replacement hormones. I have, therefore, begun prescribing an indefinite course of 0.625 mg of the estrogen Premarin for the first twenty-five days of the month, and 5 mg of the progesterone Provera for days sixteen to twenty-five. I use the antibiotic to cure the infection and the hormones to prevent reoccurrence. I tell my patients that they may talk it over with their gynecologist, but that if there are any objections I would like to know. I am impressed with my patients' improved health but concerned by the headaches experienced by a few. In these cases, halving the hormone dosage has eliminated the headaches, but whether it will continue to improve the resilience of the vagina and urethra remains to be seen.

In 1995 another study found an association between the use of estrogen and breast cancer development. The suggestion is not new. Previous studies had indicated such an association, only to be disproven or unsubstantiated by other studies. What should women do? Certainly, women with a tendency to breast cysts should avoid the hormones, as should women with a family history of breast cancer. Perhaps women who develop breast tenderness should also avoid the hormones. On the other hand, women whose lives have been improved with estrogen treatment should think twice before discontinuing the pills. It is not as if cancer is the inevitable result of estrogen therapy.

The Unstable Bladder

It is possible that your partner has symptoms of infection – a frequent, urgent desire to urinate and discomfort in the lower abdomen – and no infection at all. This is a common occurrence. Bladders develop bad habits rather quickly and easily. Thus, frequent and urgent urination, originally due to bacterial infection, may persist long after the irritating bacteria have been eliminated. Also, frequency and urgency that began with a stressful life crisis may persist long after the cause of the problem has been resolved. This frequent and urgent desire to empty the bladder, even when there are no bacteria in the urine or disease in the bladder wall, is called an unstable bladder.

I believe that our misconceptions about the nervous system contribute to our poor management of this condition. From the first mention of the nervous system, perhaps in high school, North American students learn that there are two nervous systems: the voluntary and the involuntary. We learn that we can, for example, direct a finger here or there because the muscles that guide the movement are directed by the voluntary nervous system. At the same time, we learn that organs such as the bladder are controlled by the involuntary nervous system. Apart from controlling the sphincter muscle and shutting off the flow when we have to, we are taught that the organ behaves autonomously and automatically. Thus, when the bladder develops a pattern of emptying too frequently, we cannot understand how we can use our minds to will the organ to change its behaviour. Many doctors, as well, are not so certain that the bladder can be subject to willpower. Pills are consequently prescribed to relax the contractions of the bladder muscles. And yet many patients have controlled an unstable bladder without drugs. They have methodically stretched the time intervals between urination by, perhaps, five-minute increments every day. Over a period of months, this retraining has had as good results as drugs. Asian civilizations, it seems, do not have this hang-up about the autonomic nervous system. Zen and Yoga both teach that "Yes, you can control your involuntary nervous system." Of course it is easier to prescribe a few pills, or even undertake psychotherapy.

If the patient has an unstable bladder and cannot voluntarily repattern the frequent and urgent need to urinate, the condition can normally be cured in two months by drugs. The most commonly used drug for this purpose is oxybutynin (Ditropan), at a dosage of 5 mg twice or three times a day. A very dry mouth and throat are inevitable side effects of this drug. When side effects prohibit the use of oxybutynin, I try my patients on flavoxate (Urispas), which can relax certain muscles, or dicyclomine hydrochloride (Bentylol), which is an anti-spasmodic preparation used primarily for an overactive intestine.

Hysterectomy

Surgical removal of the uterus is a procedure decided upon by gynecologists, and, as a urologist, I have no quarrel with that. But when a hysterectomy is proposed not because of any malady within the uterus, but because it may help correct urinary symptoms, I do protest. A large uterus may appear to be pressing on the roof of the bladder, but this seldom, if ever, causes urinary symptoms.

There is also a tendency to do what are thought of as "preventive" bladder operations at the same time as hysterectomies. Although the removal of the uterus *can* damage bladder and urethral supports, surgery should be undertaken only when there is an actual problem.

A hysterectomy does not affect the sexuality of most

women, but some find that orgasms become less pleasurable after removal of the uterus. Since we know that pelvic muscles contract and the uterus changes shape and position during sexual excitement and orgasm, it makes sense that the sexual experience in a woman without a uterus may be altered.

If your partner has had a hysterectomy, she may feel psychologically wounded. Extra kindness and consideration at this point will help restore normal sexual feelings.

Stress Incontinence

Stress incontinence is a frequently unmentioned, late complication of hysterectomy. Many doctors choose not to warn patients about it because incontinence may only develop years after surgery, although the loss of bladder supports during surgery is the original cause of problem. In addition to women who have had a hysterectomy, incontinence mostly affects women over fifty who smoke a lot, are overweight, or have had more than two large babies. Kegel's exercises, which strengthen the sphincter muscles, can prevent stress incontinence and treat the early cases. The patient is directed to try to stop the urine in the middle of the flow, or at least to slow it down. If she can do that, she is contracting the right muscle. Another instruction is to ask the patient to pull the buttocks together. She is directed to contract the sphincter muscles one hundred to two hundred times a day. Mild cases, or patients who are very anxious to avoid surgery, are placed on a regime of exercises and medications. The two pills that have proven useful are imipramine (Tofranil), which is an antidepressant, and decongestants such as pseudoephedrine (Sudafed). These medications act on nerve receptors located at the neck of the bladder. The muscle tone increases and resistance to outflow is improved.

Sexuality and Urinary Control

Some women cannot achieve orgasm without urinating. I have been consulted a number of times for this "problem." My advice over the years has been to protect the mattress, nothing more.

One young lady came to see me because she was still bed-wetting, at age twenty-five. She had just got engaged, and the wedding date was fast approaching. Was there a way, she asked, to correct the embarrassing problem before the wedding night? She was free of infection and had no other problems. I pre-scribed imipramine (Tofranil), the drug used for mild stress incontinence and bed-wetting in children, but I warned her that it was unlikely there would be sufficient time before the wedding for the drug to take effect.

"If you wet the bed on your wedding night," I suggested, "tell your husband that his sexual prowess and your ecstatic orgasms are responsible."

On the first day of her honeymoon she called to say, "It worked," and hung up. To this day I am not sure what worked: the medication, or the story.

My counsel in this case was an unusual solution to an extreme problem. I do not generally recommend subterfuge. I believe in a straightforward, honest approach to private-part problems. There is a fundamental difference in the anatomy and physiology of the two sexes, and I think men and women benefit from knowing the kind of health problems each may develop. Understanding gives us an added appreciation of the other and lessens misunderstanding. Obviously, the person who knows his mate's body makes a better partner.

Questions and Answers

- **Can a dipstick test be used instead of a urine culture to test for a bladder infection?**

The dipstick can provide considerable information if the urine sample is fresh and read exactly one minute after dipping. It tells whether the urine is acid or alkaline, if there is any sugar, protein, red blood cells, white blood cells, or ketones. The presence of nitrites on the stick is indirect evidence of infection. It is a good first test. But the urine culture is needed to know how infected the specimen is and what specific antibiotics are required.

- **If I walk on a cold cement floor, can that bring on a bladder infection?**

Chilled feet, exposure to a cold draft, and constipation are all clinically recognized as factors that have predisposed the bladder to infection. Why this occurs is not clear.

- **If a woman keeps using antibiotics for a chronic bladder infection, will she hurt her body?**

An allergy to a medication can develop at any time. Symptoms include dizziness, headaches, upset stomach, abdominal cramps, and skin rash. Allergies may also effect changes in the blood and are suspected in cases with a lowered white cell count or a lowered platelet count. Also, some bacteria adapt to and resist a particular antibiotic. Despite these risks, repeated long-term use of antibiotics does alleviate a chronic problem and is usually safe.

- **Can I harm myself by urinating only once or twice a day?**

Some people have naturally large bladders and do not need to evacuate often. But those who develop very large bladders by not responding to the call of nature can harm the bladder by overstretching it. This leads to non-resilient bladder muscles that have lost their ability to contract. So lax are some muscles that some women, and very rarely men, can only evacuate the bladder by inserting a catheter several times a day.

- **Can a woman get bladder symptoms because of menopause?**

A young vagina is about thirty cells thick, while an older vagina may thin to about six cells thick. If the older vagina is dry, sore, and itchy, as well as thin, it is suffering from atrophic vaginitis. These vaginal changes do not cause urethral or bladder irritation, but similar changes occur in the urethra and can cause symptoms. These vaginal and urethral changes are largely due to a lack of estrogen and can be reversed by replacement hormones.

- **Can a person get a bladder transplant?**

A bladder transplant from one person into another is never done, because a new bladder can be made from parts of the small or large intestine. It is a major undertaking but can be quite successful.

- **If a woman has surgery to correct stress incontinence will it affect her sexual enjoyment?**

Surgery to correct stress incontinence applies stitches to the so-called G-spot, located on the front wall of the vagina about

10 cm (4 inches) from the outside. This area is not scientifically established as a female erogenous zone, but even if it were, sensation should not be affected since the nerves are not damaged in surgery.

- **What is a partial hysterectomy?**

Surgical removal of the uterus without removal of the cervix is called a partial hysterectomy. This operation used to be done with the intention of reducing damage to the ureter and bladder. Now doctors feel that no woman should consent to a partial hysterectomy, as the tissue of the cervix is prone to cancer formation.

- **Can a woman have a hysterectomy through the vagina rather than through the lower abdomen?**

A woman can state her preference, but the best approach depends upon the shape of the pelvis or the condition of the uterus.

Pelvises can be wide-necked or narrow-necked. If the pelvis is wide-necked, a vaginal hysterectomy is possible; if the pelvis is too narrow, doing the hysterectomy through the vagina can damage the urinary tract.

If a hysterectomy is being done for cancer of the uterus, a lymph node dissection is necessary to stage the disease. In this case, an abdominal hysterectomy is the only choice.

- **Should a woman get a second opinion if a hysterectomy is proposed?**

Hysterectomies are done routinely for the following valid reasons:

a. cancer of the uterus, ovaries, or vagina;
b. life-threatening haemorrhage during childbirth;
c. prolapse of the uterus such that it is protruding from the vagina;
d. uncontrolled bleeding associated with a benign tumour of the uterus called a fibroid;
e. occasional cancers or life-threatening infections that have spread to the uterus.

A second opinion should be sought if a hysterectomy is proposed for any reason other than those listed above.

11

Urinary Incontinence

The years take their toll on the plumbing of an old house, the pipes often getting blocked or springing leaks. In similar fashion, an aging body places a strain on its "plumbing," often resulting in urinary retention (the inability to empty the bladder) and urinary incontinence (the involuntary loss of urine). Thirty per cent of elderly people living at home suffer incontinence, as do more than 50 per cent living in institutions. This translates into between eleven and fourteen million people in Canada and the United States suffering from incontinence, and by the year 2000, the cost of adult diapers and other protective garments will exceed six billion dollars in the United States. Women, overall, are affected twice as often as men.

So, if you are a tax-paying member of society likely to share the burden of this cost, or if you are likely to have an elderly occupant in your home, or if you have genes that are likely to provide you with a long life, understanding incontinence should prove useful and important.

The powerful smell of stagnant urine is very unpleasant. It is caused by the bacteria that break down the urea in urine into ammonia. The bacteria called *Proteus mirabilis* is the most common offender, but other bacteria can also break down urea into carbon dioxide and two molecules of ammonia. Curiously, before the invention of the microscope, when micro-organisms became visible, it was believed that ammoniacal decomposition of urine caused infection, not the other way around.

Undoubtedly it is the malodour that makes urinary incontinence such a crippling medico-social problem. Incontinence keeps otherwise healthy and alert citizens at home, away from social interaction and communal activities. It deprives its elderly victims of a welcome in the homes of acquaintances and friends, even family, and it often blocks admission into certain nursing homes and residences.

Incontinence can be continuous, like a leaky faucet that drips steadily, or intermittent, with periods of dryness. Continuous dribbling can occur when the tap muscle, or urinary sphincter, has been damaged or destroyed; when the sphincter can't open, with the bladder filling to capacity and the excess dribbling out in what is called overflow incontinence; or when the urine leaks out of a hole in the system (known as a fistula). Examples of intermittent incontinence include bed-wetting (enuresis), urgency incontinence, and stress incontinence. The different types of incontinence can overlap or occur concurrently. Doctors looking after a patient with incontinence will often request a voiding diary – detailing how much was voided how often – to help clarify the situation. In practice, doctors categorize incontinence in the following way.

Enuresis (Bed-Wetting)

Involuntary loss of urine during sleep, or bed-wetting, has the medical name enuresis. As a child matures he or she develops daytime control by the age of three, give or take a year, and nighttime control by the age of five, give or take a year. When children do not establish nighttime control by the time they start school, parents become alarmed, and their alarm increases the child's anxiety. The vast majority of children outgrow enuresis if the parents are patient. I think it unwise to institute drastic measures too soon, as it can be psychologically harmful to the child.

Treatment

As I have already suggested, children almost always outgrow enuresis, or bed-wetting. To encourage a more rapid resolution of the problem, parents should limit what the child drinks after the evening meal, ensure that the child empties his bladder at bedtime, and wake the child to go again when the parents retire. This simple regimen will cure a number of patients. In stubborn cases I prescribe imipramine (Tofranil) at a dose of 25 mg up to 75 mg at bedtime. Imipramine has side effects, but they are uncommon. When imipramine alone proves unsatisfactory, I add oxybutynin (Ditropan), the drug used to relax the muscles of the bladder. Often the combination of imipramine and oxybutynin solves the problem. Recently, a medication that depresses urine production, an anti-diuretic hormone administered as a nighttime nasal spray, has been introduced. It is called desmopressin acetate nasal spray (DDAVP for short). It does work, but I have had little experience with it. I have also had very little experience with electronic devices that give a child a mild electric shock as bed-wetting occurs. It is effective in some cases, but it can be psychologically damaging to some children.

Stress Incontinence

The "stress" in stress incontinence refers not to an emotional state but to a mechanical stress placed on the bladder by a cough, a sneeze, a jump, or a stretch. The increased pressure on the bladder is too much for the control tap.

Normally, the junction of the bladder neck and its outflow tract, the urethra, is held in position by a ligament suspended from the pubic bone. A sudden pressure on the bladder does not get transmitted to the urethra, because the ligament forms a kink of the urethra at its origin. This suspensory ligament may be stretched, damaged, or destroyed in women by the trauma of childbirth. The bladder neck and urethra will then drop from their mooring. The result is a urethrocele which results in stress incontinence, because pressure on the bladder becomes pressure on the urethra.

Diagnosis

The symptoms of stress incontinence and urgency incontinence (see page 238-39) often overlap or occur concurrently. This can lead to an error in diagnosis. It is important for the doctor to distinguish between the two types of incontinence, because corrective measures applied to one will not help the other. In particular, surgical procedures to correct stress incontinence have no application for urgency incontinence. Stress and urgency incontinence occur in both men and women, but they occur more frequently in women.

In order to minimize errors, a cystoscopic assessment, as well as elaborate tests called urodynamic studies, are undertaken.

Cystoscopy

Cystoscopy is a diagnostic test performed by a urologist. I do this test with the patient under a local anaesthetic and, as a rule, the procedure is usually much more distressing to men than to women. This is because the urethra is much longer in men than in women; 20.5 cm (about 8 inches) compared to

4 cm (about 1.5 inches). Also, women who visit a gynecologist regularly are more used to an examination of the genitals.

The patient is asked to lie flat on his back with his feet in stirrups, a position often assumed by a woman giving birth. After a wash and rinse, 5 mL of a local anaesthetic incorporated into a gel is instilled into the urinary passage from the tip of the penis. I then take the cystoscope, which I have described before as looking like a tiny telescope the width of a pencil, and slowly insert it into the passage. The insertion is done with a column of water leading the way. As the cystoscope approaches the sphincter at the neck of the bladder, the pressure on the water is not enough to maintain an open channel, and the instrument makes contact with the sphincter wall. The patient feels this, and can find it distressing and even painful. If the prostate is enlarged, there is further contact with the wall of the urethra at this point, causing more unpleasant sensations. Once the cystoscope is into the bladder, there is no discomfort. Now a urine sample is taken and the entire wall of the bladder can be examined.

When the sphincter has been damaged, I can see that it will not close even when I ask my patient to deliberately stop the flow.

Urodynamic Tests

Flow Test: Instead of voiding into a toilet, the patient empties his full bladder into a receptacle that records the amount of urine passed per unit of time. The maximum flow rate, which should exceed 15 mL/second, provides information regarding possible blockages or weaknesses in the bladder muscle. A reduced flow rate or intermittent flow is often seen in men with an enlarged and obstructing prostate gland.

Urethral Pressure Profile: In this test, a qualified lab technician, a nurse, or a doctor, passes a small catheter, perhaps 3 mm (an eighth of an inch) in diameter, into the urethra and records the pressure necessary to overcome resistance to an inflow of fluid through side holes in the tube at different levels of the urethra. A patient with a damaged sphincter will have less resistance to this inflow. This can be a valuable test, but it is not without complications, such as an infection or a scratch of the urethral wall. Also, the results are not as reproducible as other tests such as an electrocardiogram.

Cystometrogram: A catheter is inserted and the bladder filled with sterile water or with carbon dioxide. The reaction of the bladder muscle to filling is recorded. Normally the muscles of the bladder do not contract until it is near capacity, at which point it registers a series of contractions. Patients with urgency incontinence have inappropriate contractions long before capacity is reached. These are called uninhibited contractions.

Modern urodynamic laboratories offer even more elaborate tests. For example, ultrasound examinations can be made as the bladder fills or empties. Or a needle can be placed into the muscle of the anal sphincter to record voluntary muscle activity to coincide with the activity of the bladder muscle. Normally, as the bladder muscles contract, the sphincter muscle relaxes. If both muscles contract simultaneously, urination cannot occur normally.

Urodynamic studies is an evolving science. It can help clarify a complicated problem, but some urologists still pooh-pooh the tests, claiming the results are not sufficiently reproducible.

Treatment

Stress incontinence is a problem that can vary in severity, from a loss of a few drops from very strenuous activity, such as tennis or aerobic exercises, to the loss of cupfuls from normal daily activity. Obviously, the treatment should not be the same. Stress incontinence in men is much less common than it is in women, but it is becoming a more frequent problem because it often occurs after radical prostatectomy (removal of the prostate gland), which is increasingly common.

For mild stress incontinence, I ask my patient to develop the sphincter muscle by regularly exercising it. No patient is too old to increase the strength of the sphincter muscle. If he has difficulty learning how to contract the muscle, I arrange biofeedback sessions, which teach the patient the appropriate response by signalling when he is doing well. When exercise is not enough, I add imipramine (Tofranil) to the regime. Occasionally a patient will require both Tofranil and pseudo-ephedrine (Sudafed). I am not convinced that injections to increase resistance (see bovine collagen discussed on page 244) is profitable. In women, severe stress incontinence is corrected by surgery.

Urgency Incontinence

Normally there is sufficient time between the signal to void and finding a washroom. In urgency incontinence, the urge is so intense and the signal so late that there is insufficient time to deal with the underwear, let alone find a washroom.

Urgency incontinence can occur when there is a disturbance inside the bladder, like a stone or infected urine; when there is a disease in the bladder wall, like cancer, tuberculosis, or a disease called interstitial cystitis; or when there is a disorder in the nerve connection, such as may result from a stroke or cancer, that interrupts messages from the brain to the bladder. Most nerve pathways from the brain to the spinal centre for urine control dampen bladder-muscle contractions. Thus, any injury or immaturity of this pathway will result in excessive bladder contractions. In a sense, children who have not yet established control have this kind of incontinence, like an uncontrollable exaggerated knee-jerk reflex.

Diagnosis

As mentioned above, a cystoscopic assessment and urodynamic studies are undertaken to distinguish urgency and stress incontinence. These diagnostic tests are discussed on pages 235-37.

Treatment

To treat urgency incontinence, the underlying cause must be sought and addressed. For example, urgency incontinence due to a stone in the bladder or an infection can be cured by removing the stone or by treating the infection.

More often there is no obvious disease, and the only positive findings are ill-timed, excessive contractions of the bladder muscles detected on the cystometrogram. These contractions are normally suppressed, so when they occur they are called uninhibited contractions. Patients with this problem respond to bladder retraining, which is more easily achieved when an accurate voiding diary is kept. Most patients require, in addition, medications that relax the smooth muscles directly, such as flavoxate (Urispas), or indirectly through the nervous system, such as oxybutynin (Ditropan) or dicyclomine (Bentylol). Ditropan is probably the most popular drug. The effective dosage is 5 mg two to three times a day. The full dosage must be approached slowly and gradually to minimize disabling dryness of the mouth and throat. Elderly patients tolerate Ditropan poorly, and a better medication for them might be propanthelin bromide (Pro-banthine) 15 mg three times a day. The pill regime must be continued for a minimum of two months to change the behavioural pattern of the bladder.

Overflow Incontinence

In overflow incontinence the sphincter is intact but the bladder muscle cannot evacuate the bladder's content. It fills to capacity and the excess dribbles out. The bladder does not rupture unless it suffers a sudden blow when it is full.

Overflow incontinence occurs when a stone, a tumour, an enlarged prostate, or any other disturbance totally blocks the bladder outlet. It can also occur when there is damage to the nerve supplying the bladder (caused by a stroke, for example), or when there is sustained overstretching of the bladder muscle (caused by not responding to the call of nature, for example). Telephone operators who were not allowed to leave their post while on duty often overstretched their bladders. And such overstretched muscles lose their capacity to contract.

Diagnosis

Overflow incontinence should, theoretically, be easy to diagnose. A full and distended bladder can be seen, felt, or tapped out in most people. In a very obese patient, however, even a very full bladder can be hidden under a mountain of fat.

Treatment

Treatment of overflow incontinence is relatively simple. The physical or structural impediment to the flow, such as an

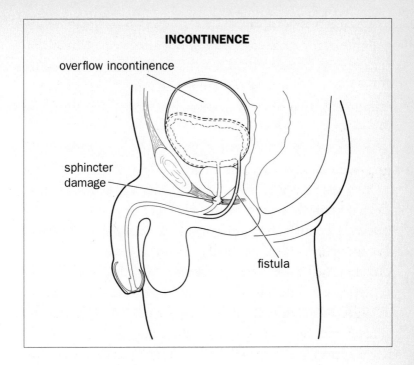

INCONTINENCE

overflow incontinence

sphincter
damage

fistula

enlarged and obstructing prostate gland, a stone, or a stricture, is eliminated. When the obstruction has been of long standing, the bladder muscles have been overstretched, and removing the obstruction does not alone solve the problem. The bladder has to be relieved with regular self-evacuation with a catheter, or by the insertion of a drainage tube from the lower abdomen into the bladder until the bladder muscles function normally again. I have seen flabby bladders recover after more than one year of treatment by periodic self-evacuation with a catheter.

Total Incontinence

In total incontinence, urine spills outside its normal tract through a fistula, or it leaks out from its normal opening because the sphincter is damaged or destroyed.

A vesico-vaginal fistula, affecting only women, is an example of the former, the urine spilling out of a hole in the bladder to empty into the vagina. Incontinence after prostate surgery is an example of the latter, the urine leaking through a tap muscle that has been damaged or destroyed.

Diagnosis

The diagnosis of total incontinence does not seem particularly difficult at first glance. How can one miss a diagnosis of urine escaping outside its normal tract? In fact it is not always so simple. I recall a little boy whose incontinence baffled a number of doctors. He urinated in a normal pattern, but he was also continually wet. The problem was traced to a small extra kidney unit that drained into his urethra instead of the bladder.

Total incontinence due to a damaged sphincter can be difficult to diagnose in women. The sphincter in a woman is not as distinct a structure as it is in a man. Urologists are forever puzzled by the female urethra. Where is the sphincter, and how do women retain urine at all?

Treatment

A continuous leak from an opening outside the normal urinary tract is a mechanical problem. The leak simply needs to be patched. Sometimes a repair is not possible, however. The leak might be from tissue that has been irradiated or filled with cancer. In these circumstances, an entire kidney with its leaking drainage system might be removed. Or, if the leak is at or below the level of the bladder, the urine might be diverted into an isolated segment of small intestine, closed at one end, and opened to the skin at the other end. A bag is worn over the opening in the skin. This is called an Ileal loop, or the Bricker procedure after the doctor who popularized it.

The resistance to the flow at the sphincter level can be

lessened by paralyzing a control nerve with a local anaesthetic. A permanent effect can be obtained by substituting absolute alcohol or phenol for the local anaesthetic.

When urine leaks out of the normal opening because the sphincter has been damaged or destroyed, a solution is even more difficult. Sometimes, when the leak is not pronounced, an attempt might be made to achieve a better balance between the forces of retention and the powers of expulsion. The expulsive forces can be diminished, for example, by increasing the size of the bladder by adding to it a segment of small intestine. The expulsive force can also be dampened by the drug Ditropan.

Sphincter resistance can be augmented by adding a substance to create a partial blockage. At one time Teflon paste was used for this purpose, but the product is no longer used, because, on occasions, Teflon particles migrated to the lungs. Today a product called bovine collagen, made from the tissue of cows, is used instead. The product is injected so that it lies just under the inner lining of the urethra at its origin. A number of patients are allergic to this very expensive product. The patient's own fat cells have been tried for this purpose, but the effects are not long-lasting.

When all else fails, an artificial sphincter is considered. Developed largely by the late Dr. Brantley Scott, of Houston, Texas, the artificial sphincter works on the same principle as a cuff used to measure blood pressure. The inflatable portion of the apparatus is wrapped around the bladder neck or urethra. When the cuff is filled, the patient is dry; when emptied, the urine drains out. In theory, the artificial sphincter works fine. In practice there are problems with leakages when the pressure in the cuff is not high enough, and with erosion of the apparatus into the urinary tract when the pressure is too high. I believe that an ideal artificial sphincter could work on a much lower pressure and sit just inside the urinary lining above the muscle layer of the bladder. It awaits development. In the meantime another last resort is to use either condom drainage or a Cunningham clamp. In the former method, the patient wears a regular condom, the tip of which opens to a rubber tube that is connected to a drainage bag. The Cunningham clamp is like a padded clothespin applied to the shaft of the penis. It has solved the problem for some patients, but has created complications, such as pressure injury, in others.

Questions and Answers

- **Why is the management of incontinence with adult diapers considered better than a catheter and bag?**

A patient using diapers is unlikely to develop urine infection, whereas catheter patients will always have urinary infections.

- **Can collagen injections be used in men with incontinence after the prostate has been surgically removed?**

There is no good reason why it cannot be tried. Injection treatment has been far less successful in men than in women.

- **Can stress incontinence occur in men?**

It is very rare, except in men whose prostate has been removed.

- **Is there a way to neutralize the bad smell of urine?**

There are preservative tablets that may inhibit normal urine odour. Ammonia odour cannot be suppressed.

- **What is the best product to minimize urine irritation in incontinent patients?**

One brand of barrier cream is much the same as another.

- **Is it inevitable that as I age I will have to run more and more often to the washroom and will leak more and more?**

By and large, this is true, but, whenever possible, incontinence or the need to urinate frequently should be treated.

12

Urinary Tract Infection

Some fifty years ago, many thought that the new anti-microbial agents (the sulfonamides, penicillin, and other antibiotics) heralded the end of bacterial diseases such as pneumonia, meningitis, and urinary tract infections, in the same way that vaccination wiped out smallpox. Alas, how wrong they were! Vaccination did eliminate smallpox, by and large, but anti-microbial agents did not eradicate bacterial infections. Instead, their production launched a multi-billion dollar industry, achieving, at best, some containment of the problem.

A urinary tract infection (UTI) is a bacterial infection of the kidney, bladder, prostate, or urethra. The bacteria get into the urinary tract at the exit, the meatus, and from the urethra they climb up through the system. I have touched on this subject before in different parts of this book: prostate infection or prostatitis in Chapter 4, bladder infection or cystitis in Chapter 10, and urethral infection or urethritis in Chapter 8.

UTI is a common problem, accounting for six million treated cases per year in the United States, with yearly costs in excess of a billion dollars. You might not be aware, however, of the slick sales campaign waged by the pharmaceutical companies to capture a share of the market. This chapter may help you decide whether you are getting the best advice from your beleaguered practitioner.

The Patient

A baby boy is susceptible to UTI because of the colonization of bacteria under the foreskin. Boys circumcised at birth have UTI four times less often. Middle-aged men get prostatitis (prostate infection), often associated with UTI. Older men with prostate enlargement or prostate cancer often get UTI, related to an incomplete evacuation of the bladder on urination.

Pre-school-age girls get UTI more often than boys because the short urethra in females makes them more vulnerable. Sexually active women are vulnerable because the bacteria that have colonized the skin near the vagina get delivered into the bladder. Pregnant women are vulnerable for reasons not totally clear, and post-menopausal women get UTI because they lose the protection provided by estrogen.

The Diagnosis

The diagnosis of UTI is based on the patient's history, on an examination of the patient, and on examination of the urine. But symptoms and laboratory reports can, at times, lead the doctor astray.

A patient will typically come to his doctor complaining of burning, a frequent and urgent need to urinate, lower-abdominal pain, and perhaps some lower-back pain. These classic symptoms of bladder infection are also the symptoms of: genito-urinary tuberculosis; a particular form of bladder cancer called carcinoma-in-situ; a bladder disorder called interstitial cystitis; and a bladder stone.

The examination of the patient is important because it is

useful to distinguish between a kidney infection and a bladder infection, and elaborate schemes have been proposed to distinguish between the two. The duration of treatment is drastically different: treatment for bladder infection can be three days; the treatment for kidney infection may be two to six weeks. In kidney infection, the pain is high in the back, there is tenderness to a punch over the kidney, and there is likely to be fever and chills. The urine may show characteristic barlike clumps, called casts, containing remnants of white blood cells.

Laboratory confirmation of a kidney infection can be expensive and potentially hazardous. For example, urine samples collected directly from the kidney can be tested, a procedure requiring cystoscopy and the passing of a small hollow tube up to the kidney to collect the urine, which can cause an infection. This urine can be examined for: the telltale presence of antibody-coated white blood cells (although unfortunately this test is not living up to its early promise and has been abandoned in most centres); an elevated level of certain iso-enzymes in the urine such as Lactic DeHydrogenase (LDH); and signs that the kidney is unable to concentrate urine adequately. The urine might also be tested after the bladder has been washed out to eliminate any effects it might have on the results.

A dipstick examination of the urine can provide clues as to whether an infection is present. Different spots on the strip denote the presence of sugar, protein, acidity, red blood cells, white blood cells, and bacteria. The dip-stick does not indicate the amount of bacteria or its identity.

A urine sample collected in mid-stream and tested to see how many colonies of bacteria will grow from 1 mL (known as a quantitative mid-stream culture) remains an excellent test for kidney infection. Bacteria that spill into the urine at the kidney level inoculate the innocent bladder, where they sit and multiply, doubling their numbers every twenty minutes and reaching figures of 100,000 and more.

A quantitative urine culture is unnecessary for simple bladder infections acquired in the community, but a culture should be done for complicated infections acquired in hospitals, or whenever the kidney is involved. Urine for culture can be obtained by sticking a needle into the bladder from a puncture site in the lower abdomen. There is considerable resistance to this technique, which I find difficult to understand. Why ask medical students and nurses to stick wide-bore needles into tiny veins and then tell them to avoid a target the size of an orange? A spinal needle hurts no more than a needle for blood tests. A bacterial count of 2,000 or more from such a sample is considered significant for patients who have symptoms. The kind of bacteria isolated is also important. The bacteria that cause cystitis often have one hundred to two hundred filaments or tentacles covering their surface. These filaments permit the bacteria to stick to different surfaces, like the anal area, vagina, urethra, and bladder.

The Treatment

Anti-microbial agents are used to treat UTI. The doctor must choose the appropriate agent from a wide list of available drugs and decide how long the treatment should last. Some doctors will stick with a drug that has served them well for decades, and will not try any others no matter how many new preparations have hit the market. Others will want to try the latest and newest product, feeling that they are providing the most up-to-date care. I shall state what I do in my own practice. What I recommend today, though, may not be what I recommend tomorrow. Perhaps there is merit in the adage: "Be not the first by whom the new are tried, nor yet the last to lay the old aside."

Advice on general measures vary somewhat from doctor to doctor and range from Grandma's time-tested formula to herbal medicine and witchcraft. There is no particular diet, exercise, herb, or preparation to minimize risks of acquiring a UTI, although constipation may be a factor and a high-fibre diet to prevent constipation may be wise. Getting chilled and remaining in a wet bathing suit are also unwise.

Fluid intake is another matter. Urologists like to encourage high water intake. A urologist friend of mine can say "drink lots of water" in twelve different languages. It's the most important message we can broadcast, he says, and I don't doubt that patients feel better when they drink plenty of water when they are fighting a UTI. Passing dilute urine is less painful and less distressing than passing concentrated urine. But does it help the patient? Can you flush out the bacteria? I doubt it. The bacteria, as I have said, stick to the walls of the urinary tract, and all the flushing in the world is not going to wash them off. In fact, urea, the waste product of protein breakdown, kills bacteria in normal concentration, whereas dilute urine contains too little. Still, keeping the patient comfortable is more important, and drinking lots of fluids definitely helps in this respect.

Cranberry juice *is* magical. It was long believed that the hippuric acid in the juice created enough acidity to destroy bacteria, but the amount of acidity in two glasses of the juice is not nearly enough to harm bacteria. It has been determined, though, that cranberry juice stops bacteria from sticking to the wall of the bladder. This anti-adhesive quality cannot be attributed to the juice's content of hippuric acid, ascorbic acid, or fructose, its three main ingredients. It may be the peculiar *combination* of the three ingredients or other unidentified chemicals that give it its magical quality. Some people find the commercial cocktail too sweet, and cranberry capsules, available in health-food stores may be taken instead.

What about the choice of antibiotics when the problem is a complicated hospital-acquired UTI? The choice of an appropriate agent or agents will be determined by the urine and blood culture results. These results normally take forty-eight to seventy-two hours, because they depend upon growing bacteria on a gelatin plate and testing how different antibiotics inhibit the growth. Thus, treatment is started as soon as the specimens for the laboratory have been collected. The popular treatment during the past twenty-five years has been the combination of an aminoglycoside antibiotic, such as gentamicin, netilmycin, or tobramycin, combined with ampicillin. This regime has been challenged in recent years by the third-generation cephalosporins, and even more recently – because of difficulty killing the bacteria known as pseudomonas – by the quinolones, such as ciprofloxacin, norfloxacin, or ofloxacin, all of which can be taken by mouth. After forty-eight hours or more of such treatment, the drug regime suggested by the culture results are prescribed for a minimum of two weeks.

It is for the simple, community-acquired bladder infection that there is the widest choice of preparations, and where pharmaceutical salespeople may most affect a doctor's choice. Of the six million cases of UTI diagnosed annually in the United States, five million are simple infections.

I use the trimethoprim-sulfamethoxazole combination (Septra or Bactrim) most often, nitrofurantoin (Macrodantin) when there is a known allergy to sulfonamides, and the quinolones (Noroxin, Cipro, or Floxin) when the attacks are severe or recurrent. When I prescribe the quinolones I make certain a female patient is not pregnant. For pregnant women the only good choice is a penicillin (Amoxil), although secondary yeast infection can occur.

Controversy remains regarding the length of treatment. Recommended treatment for simple infection has changed from two weeks to ten days, to seven days, to a six-pills-at-once regime. Now the most popular regime is three days.

Complicated infection involving the kidney is too often inadequately treated, in my estimation. Two weeks of treatment, the usual recommendation in medical textbooks, is not enough. In experimental studies of pyelonephritis, bacterial remnants persist in the kidney for five and six weeks.

The inner part of the kidney is an unusual environment for bacteria and it favours those without cell walls, the so-called L-forms of bacteria. It is also an environment that inhibits the natural defence mechanisms whereby bacteria are gobbled up by wandering white blood cells and where an environment wherein immune reactions are inactivated. I thus have no qualms about recommending six weeks of drug treatment when the kidneys are involved in a UTI. I would rather err on the side of overtreatment than undertreatment for this condition.

Usually, discussions of UTI exclude mention of prostatitis (infection of the prostate) and urethritis (infection of the urethra), although the prostatic urethra and the urethra constitute part of the urinary tract.

Prostatitis has been discussed in Chapter 4, on the prostate. Routine urine culture (and blood culture) can help diagnose acute prostatitis but cannot rule in or rule out the diagnosis of chronic prostatitis. Not long ago a young man suffering from impotence came to me for a second opinion. His urologist had tried to treat him, with no success. Finally, he had suggested a penile prosthesis. It turned out the young man had chronic bacterial prostatitis. He had all the classic findings, but the loss of erection was so devastating (he was into a new relationship) the other symptoms seemed inconsequential. Treatment of his prostatitis restored his potency.

Urethritis has been discussed, in part, in Chapter 8, on sexually transmitted diseases. In the past all non-gonorrheal urethritis was called non-specific urethritis (NSU). Today we recognize most cases of NSU as being caused by chlamydia. Routine urine culture cannot diagnose gonorrhea or chlamydia. Scrapings from the urethra 1 cm (.4 inches) from the meatus must be sent to a laboratory to be tested for chlamydia, and a smear of the discharge to be tested for gonorrhea. If the tests are done sloppily there can be a false negative result (that is, the disease is present, but the test negative) with delayed treatment for the patient. If the urethral scraping is done too vigorously it can be quite painful and result in bleeding, scarring, and stricture formation. A urine test for chlamydia has recently been developed. It is most welcome.

A Final Word

UTI is common and usually causes obvious symptoms, but it can be missed, because the disease may also be present without any symptoms at all. Like most medical problems, an early diagnosis and prompt treatment assures successful elimination of the offending bacteria.

Questions and Answers

- **Under what circumstances are urine cultures unnecessary in dealing with a UTI?**

Three categories of urinary tract infection are recognized: acute uncomplicated UTI, acute uncomplicated kidney infection, and complicated UTI. In an acute uncomplicated UTI, urine cultures may not be necessary.

- **What is meant by a complicated UTI?**

When urinary tract infection is associated with concurrent disorders of the kidney, obstruction, stones, foreign bodies, or inadequate or inappropriate previous treatments, we have what is called a complicated UTI.

- **Can I cure a UTI with plenty of cranberry juice?**

Cranberry juice can inhibit the development of a UTI but cannot cure an established infection.

- **Should a person with an indwelling catheter be on antibiotics?**

Any person with an indwelling catheter that drains into an open receptacle will have infection within forty-eight hours. If the drainage is into a closed system, the infection rate is 50 per cent in two weeks. Thus, whenever indwelling catheters can be avoided, as by intermittent catheterization, the patient is better off.

Whenever a patient with an indwelling catheter has infection with symptoms, each episode requires a course of antibacterials. The frequent use of antibiotics or antibacterials to prevent infection invites the emergence of resistant bacteria. Sometimes antibacterials are used as a preventive because an infection can be catastrophic and resistant organisms might be the lesser of two evils.

- **Are antibacterial agents used too much because of the pushy sales pitch of the pharmaceutical industry?**

Undoubtedly, there is this risk. The common errors are the use of antibacterials when there are irritative symptoms but no infection, and not prescribing a long-enough treatment when the infection is in the kidney or prostate.

- **Why is the three-day treatment considered better than a single dose treatment in a simple UTI?**

The recurrence rate is less frequent.

- **Do all UTIs promote kidney stones?**

Infections with bacteria that split urea into ammonia promote a urine medium favourable for a particular kind of kidney stone. Proteus is the most common urea-splitting organism.

Any kidney stone that obstructs the flow of urine can promote UTI.

- **Can UTIs be affected by diets?**

Diets to promote or discourage UTI have little basis in science.

- **Can a UTI be passed on to a sexual partner?**

Kidney and bladder infections cannot, and neither can prostatitis. Urethritis, categorized more as a sexually transmitted
disease than a UTI, can certainly be passed on by sexual
contact.

- **Can a person make a complete recovery from a kidney
  infection or will there always be a degree of kidney
  damage?**

The recovery can be so complete that tests to assess kidney
function and isotope studies can detect no change. But an
infection *can* cause lasting damage to kidney function and
changes in the isotope studies.

13

Above the Private Parts: Disorders of the Kidney

"Are you telling me every single athlete has blood in his urine after playing a contact sport like football or hockey?" asked my friend.

"If we're talking about minute amounts of blood not visible to the naked eye, yes, I think that's so," I replied.

"Where does this blood come from?"

"From the kidney, although a jogger can get bloody urine if he runs on an empty bladder. The blood is apparently due to one wall of the bladder rubbing against the opposite wall. A glass or two of water before the run to 'lubricate' the bladder eliminates the problem."

My friend was not a runner, and my little piece of advice on how to avoid a jogger's bladder did not impress him.

"Why does the kidney bleed so easily?" he asked, persisting with our original topic.

"I don't think anybody knows for sure. For me, the more tantalizing question is why bleeding from the kidney doesn't occur more often and more profusely. Did you know 25 per cent of all the blood pumped out of the heart goes straight to the kidneys? That's a lot of blood for the kidneys to process, and an enormous source, don't you think, for a little spillage.

"Furthermore," I continued, "the kidneys are held in their position – under the rib cage behind the abdomen, and in front of the back muscles – by nothing more than a pad of fat. There's no supporting tissue to anchor them to solid structures the way muscles are fixed to bone, for example, or the way other organs like the spleen, liver, or gut are suspended by ligaments. And the kidneys aren't contained within a protective cage, like the lung or the heart. They float about in the breeze, so to speak, in a soft cushion of fat."

A generation or two ago, doctors often made the colourful diagnosis of "floating" kidneys. They used to think an excessive movement of the organ could cause the drainage pipe to kink upon itself and cause pain like that experienced with a kidney stone. A severe attack, called Dietel's Crisis, was viewed as an indication for a surgical correction. Surprisingly, the diagnosis is seldom, if ever, made today. Human anatomy has not changed, it's the doctors' perception that has changed.

The kidneys are organs high above the private parts, as much as a forearm's length away. But they are connected by a long pipe called the ureter, which takes the urine from the kidneys, where it is made, to the bladder, where it is stored. The kidneys are responsible for controlling the acidity and balance of body fluids. They do so by varying salt combinations and the amount of water retained and expelled by the body.

As a urologist, I operate on the kidney, removing it or excising part of it when there is disease in the organ, repairing it if there has been an injury, or unblocking the drainage system if there is an obstruction. A urologist may also be called upon to operate on the adrenal glands, because they sit right on top of each kidney and a urologist is the surgeon most familiar with the territory. Some urologists operate on the blood vessels of the kidneys, while others prefer to leave that task to vascular surgeons.

A urologist is a surgeon-specialist of the kidney, whereas a nephrologist is a physician-specialist of the kidney. The difference lies more in what they do than in what they know. This dichotomy pervades the medical world: we have cardiovascular surgeons and cardiologists, lung surgeons and chest physicians, bowel surgeons and gastroenterologists, neurosurgeons and neurologists. There are seldom battles over territory; one specialist avidly seeks the help of the other, like having offensive and defensive players on the same team.

For kidney diseases that can be treated by drugs, changes in the diet, or changes in lifestyle, a patient should see a nephrologist. When the kidney has to be probed by an instrument or requires surgery, the patient must be seen by a urologist.

The disorders of the kidney I shall discuss in this chapter include kidney injury, diseases of the artery to the kidney, cysts on the kidney and cysts inside the kidney, cancers, stones, blockage, disorders of the filters, kidney failure, dialysis, and, finally, kidney transplantation.

Kidney Injury

As I mentioned earlier, a mild blow to the kidney can cause a microscopic blood leak into the urine. When the blow is more severe, the kidney can be torn. This can result in a collection of blood just outside the kidney. Unless the blood loss is catastrophic, the best treatment is blood transfusion and bed rest. Even if the tear results in very bloody urine, the patient is often better off being treated conservatively, as attempts to repair an injury often result in more loss of kidney substance and even total loss of the injured organ. When the blood

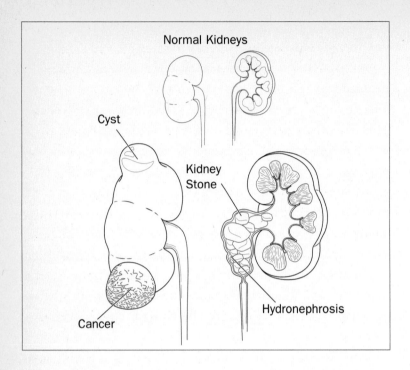

Normal Kidneys

Cyst

Kidney
Stone

Hydronephrosis

Cancer

pressure cannot be maintained with adequate transfusions, however, surgical intervention is necessary.

When the injury is due to a penetrating object, like a knife-blade or a bullet, surgery is more often undertaken, partly because infection is likely. I remember being called into the operating room to assist in treating a gunshot wound. The bullet had entered the abdomen near the belly button, gone through the large intestine, and lodged near the left kidney. Upon exploration, we found that the bullet had pierced the renal vein leaving a 2.5 (1 inch) tear on both its front and back wall. This patient lost his kidney but survived the injury. The time interval between the injury and the control of the blood vessel was about one and a half hours. But you might wonder how, with a major tear in a vein that handles more than 10 per cent of the blood circulation, the patient did not bleed out within minutes. The reason is twofold: an injury like this causes spasm of the renal artery, reducing blood flow to the kidney, and the collection of blood within the fat-cushion blocks further spillage. This patient came to see me a month later. He looked great. Indeed he was so unlike the cadaverous body on the operating table, I did not recognize him.

Renal Artery Disease and High Blood Pressure

Ten per cent of the adult population of North America has hypertension; that is, blood pressure readings above 140 over 90. It is the second reading, the diastolic, that is considered the more important; the upper, systolic, reading too often reflects the nervous tension of the moment. When the diastolic reading is over 95, medication to lower blood pressure is usually prescribed.

In 90 per cent of people with high blood pressure, the cause is unknown and the condition is called essential hypertension. "Essential hypertension" is a medical euphemism for "essentially unknown." Mild hypertension in this large population is treated by restricting salt intake and in reducing excess body weight. When the diastolic pressure remains over 95, however, drug treatment is commenced. A diuretic such as hydrochlorothiazide might be the first drug prescribed. A patient taking the pill will expel more urine, reducing the fluid in the body, including blood volume, and thus lowering the blood pressure. A beta-blocker such as propranolol (Inderal) might be added next. This family of pills, now approaching a dozen varieties, relaxes the muscle wall of the arteries and consequently lowers the blood pressure. When the blood pressure remains too high, stronger medications such as methyldopa (Aldomet) or guanethidine (Ismelin) may have to be added. As indicated in Chapter 2, most of these medications to lower blood pressure can cause impotence. When impotence can be directly related to blood pressure pills, it may help to switch to calcium channel-blockers such as diltiazem (Cardizem) or nifedipine (Adalat), or one of the angiotensin converting enzyme (ACE) inhibitors that are now in widespread use, such as captopril (Capoten) or enalapril (Vasotec). These two types of drugs, calcium channel-blockers and ACE inhibitors, are rapidly becoming established as first-line drugs, as they are well tolerated and associated less with impaired potency.

Of the remaining 10 per cent of cases of high blood pressure, half are due to hormonal imbalances from diseases of the adrenal gland. The other half are due to diseases of the kidney, resulting in equal proportions from disturbances in the kidney substance (such as stone disease, infection, cysts, and tumours, as well as diseases of the kidney filter or tubules) and diseases of the kidney artery. Thus, the condition called renovascular hypertension, where the disorder is in the kidney artery, accounts for just 2.5 per cent of the total number of patients with hypertension.

Still, this is a sizable number of patients, and the condition is worthy of discussion because this hypertension is reversible if diagnosed early enough.

Before experiments conducted by Goldblatt in 1932, it was widely held that high blood pressure damaged blood vessels, which in turn restricted blood flow. Goldblatt proved for the first time that it was the other way around: a restricted blood flow to the kidney due to diseases in the renal artery causes hypertension. The restricted blood flow released something into the bloodstream that in turn created the elevation in blood pressure. Years later the chemical substance responsible for the high blood pressure was determined. This product was an enzyme called renin, released from a particular cell within the kidney. Now drugs to counteract this, such as captopril

(Capoten) and enalapril (Vasotec), from the family of drugs called angiotensin converting enzyme (ACE) inhibitors, have been developed.

Renal Cysts

Renal cysts are liquid-filled blisters that can be on the surface or in the substance of the kidney. They can be single or multiple, and vary in size from a cherry pit to a large cantaloupe. As ultrasound examination of the abdomen is done more and more often, renal cysts are more frequently diagnosed. As many as 10 per cent of the population has cysts on the kidney. A simple cyst on the surface of the kidney, no matter how large, seldom causes symptoms or trouble. Annual monitoring with ultrasound examination is sufficient. Rarely, a giant cyst, about the size of a cantaloupe or larger, can cause some discomfort or compress adjacent organs. In these circumstances, the cyst is punctured with a needle through the skin, the fluid evacuated, and a scarring chemical, such as atabrine or absolute alcohol, instilled. It doesn't always work, but is worth trying.

Of greater concern are three other types of cysts: the parapelvic cyst, polycystic kidney disease, and the complicated cyst.

Parapelvic Cysts

A parapelvic cyst is a simple cyst in an awkward position. It lies just where the major vessels attach to the kidney and where the urine drains out of the kidney. Doctors are more reluctant to puncture a cyst in this location for fear of injuring the vessels. And when this cyst enlarges, it can block the normal drainage. On a few occasions I have had to drain this kind of cyst with surgical exploration.

Polycystic Disease

Polycystic disease is a genetic disorder of the kidney, transmitted from one generation to another as a simple dominant gene. When one parent is affected, there is a one-in-two chance that the child will inherit the disorder. In this condition, there are multiple cysts, not only on the surface of the kidney but throughout the organ. At birth the cysts are tiny, but they grow with time. The trouble starts in middle age, when the enlarging cysts begin to destroy normal kidney cells, and eventually the kidneys look like a giant sponge. Often there is bleeding into one of the larger cysts. When these patients reach their late forties or fifties, they frequently end up requiring dialysis and kidney transplantation. But, as the disease surfaces only in middle age, the problem has usually been passed on by then to the next generation.

Complicated Cysts

A complicated cyst differs from a simple cyst in having partitions within it or having calcium deposits on its wall. This kind of cyst can be due to a cancer. A simple cyst that has been injured and has perhaps filled with blood can have the same appearance, so the clinician has a difficult job choosing the correct treatment. In the hospital where I work, such cases are presented to the entire staff and a consensus is reached on how to proceed; whether we wait and monitor the problem or operate. We have not always been right. In recent years, a CT scan done in a special way with dye injection, called a dynamic CT scan, has helped clarify the diagnosis.

Cancer

Different kinds of cancers arise from the kidney. One, called Wilm's Tumour, occurs almost exclusively in children, although it can also be found, very rarely, in the young adult. Surgical removal followed by radiotherapy or chemotherapy has a 90 per cent cure rate.

Another peculiar tumour that arises from the kidney is called angiomyolipoma. It can grow and bleed, but it never spreads to other parts of the body and is thus considered benign. Years ago, when we routinely removed this growth, whenever the pathology report revealed it to be an angiomyolipoma, we would happily rush the report to the patient. Today, the CT scan can ascertain this diagnosis with confidence because of the characteristic high fat-content of the tumour. When the tumour is less than 7 cm (3 inches) or so and not causing symptoms, many doctors choose simply to keep an eye on it with periodic CT scans, and suggest surgery only if the tumour is growing out of hand with, perhaps, bleeding into it.

Tumours can also arise from the urinary lining within the kidney or kidney pelvis (the small sac in which urine sits momentarily before it drains down the pipe to empty into the bladder). The lining of the urinary tract from kidney to bladder is composed entirely of the same type of cells, so this kind of tumour is identical to those arising from the bladder. Tumours that start in the kidney, pelvis, or ureter are somewhat worse than tumours that occur first in the bladder. This is because the wall of the urinary tract is thinner *above* the bladder and a tumour there can spread out more easily. This type of tumour, called transitional cell carcinoma (TCC), is discussed below.

Transitional Cell Carcinoma (TCC)

An enormous body of information has been gathered regarding the common cancer called TCC, which manifests first with bloody urine unaccompanied by any pain. It is the fifth most-common form of cancer in men, constituting 7 per cent of all newly diagnosed cancers. The disease is less common in women, the male-to-female ratio being 3:1. We have learned that heavy exposure to rubber, leather, plastic, paint, coal, printing ink, and textile dyes increase the risk of getting TCC. So does smoking, because 2-naphthylamine and nitrosamines, chemicals present in cigarette smoke, promote bladder cancers. We have learned to predict the seriousness of the disease by the cancer's stage (how advanced it is) when it is discovered, and by the grade (how aggressive the cancer cells appear under the microscope). TCC is staged as A when the surface lining alone is involved, B when the muscle layer is invaded, C when the disease has spread beyond the muscle but is still confined to the site of origin, and D when there is widespread disease. The growth can be removed with instruments passed through the urethra when the disease has not yet spread beyond the middle depth of the muscle layer.

After removal of the growth or growths, reoccurrences in the bladder can be rendered less likely with drug treatment. A drug, such as BCG (bacillus of Calmette and Guerin), used to immunize the population against tuberculosis, is instilled into the bladder once a week for six weeks. BCG might be the most effective treatment, but other drugs that can be used include mitomycin (Mutamycin), doxorubicin (Adriamycin), and interferon alfa-2b (Intron-A).

Sometimes a portion of the bladder or the entire bladder must be removed. When the entire bladder is removed, the patient must live the rest of his life with a permanent urine bag, or learn to insert a hollow tube at regular intervals to empty an artificial bladder made from an intestinal segment.

Radiotherapy and intravenous chemotherapy are also used to treat advanced TCC. Although treatment protocols are becoming more and more standardized, we can not yet test as accurately as for bacterial infections to help choose the most appropriate drug regime.

Every urologist has his share of patients with TCC. I have patients who have never had a reoccurrence of bladder cancer but come regularly for an annual cystoscopy. Several have had numerous separate reoccurrences, some with more than fifty. Patients with reoccurrences are more fortunate, though, than those whose tumours developed deep roots and became invasive.

Toxic intravenous chemotherapy does not always work, but it can. One of my favourite patients is a woman whose original tumour was the size of a tangerine, with roots well into the bladder muscle and the tissue beyond the bladder. Surgical removal was not a realistic consideration, but cis-platinum-based chemotherapy has totally eradicated the cancer. I can still see the area where the cancer originated, but, six years later, there are no signs of disease. Another patient has had over sixty reoccurrences of bladder tumours, some in the lower segments of the ureter. Numerous removals of these tumours accompanied by various chemotherapy drug administrations into the bladder have kept her well, and she has not had reoccurrences in the last three years.

Renal Cell Carcinoma

A solid tumour arising from a kidney cell is called renal cell carcinoma. It is the most common and the most lethal kidney cancer. The life history of this tumour is one of the most unusual, most unpredictable of all the cancers. Some tumours produce a hormone that stimulates the production of excess red blood cells, others produce a hormone that raises the blood's calcium level to dangerous heights. Some of these cancers spread only to the brain, lung, or bone, without deposits anywhere else in the body. Some tumours spread directly into the venous system, so that a clot of tumour cells can extend all the way from the kidney into the heart. Sometimes heroic operations to remove such tumours and their tentacles reaching into the heart chambers can cure the patient. Surgical removal is the only worthwhile treatment, because radiotherapy and chemotherapy are ineffective for this cancer. One of my patients who had a tumour extension into the heart had to have her blood pumped artificially while her heart was stopped and the tumour removed, but she is cancer-free five years later and is back to skiing.

Fortunately the diagnosis is now being made earlier by ultrasound, before symptoms of the more advanced disease appear. The three classic signs of this cancer are bloody urine without pain and a discernible lump and pain in the area of the tumour. The tumour is staged best by the TNM method, (T for tumour, N for nodes, and M for metastases, meaning lesions that have spread). In stage 1 the tumour is confined to the substance of the kidney; in stage 2 the tumour has extended outside the capsule of the kidney but is still within the fat pad in which the kidney lies; in stage 3 the tumour has spread into the venous outflow of the kidney or into adjacent lymph nodes; and in stage 4 there are lesions that have spread beyond the nearby lymph nodes. The staging is somewhat academic and less meaningful than for prostate or bladder cancer, because no worthwhile treatment exists for the advanced disease. Whether surgery should be carried out in the presence of metastatic disease is controversial. Some experts believe that such intervention seldom if ever prolongs life or adds to the quality of life. Others argue that metastatic lesions have abated with the removal of the primary lesion often enough to offer some hope to the patient. Furthermore, they argue, a large tumour that is left alone inevitably causes massive bleeding and pain.

Recently, some inroads have been made in treating kidney cancers that have spread to distant sites. At the National Cancer Institute, in Maryland, Steven Rosenberg led a team that explored the use of biological products manufactured artificially, by a form of genetic engineering. So far, inter-leukin-2 (IL-2), tumour-infiltrating lymphocyte (TIL), and lymphokine-activated killer cells (LAK) have had limited trials with remarkable responses in 10 to 30 per cent of cases.

Why have genetically engineered products (or "magic bullets") not had a more dramatic impact on cancer therapy? The idea seems simple enough: obtain some cancer cells, inac-tivate them, then reintroduce them in such a way that the patient's body might make antibodies against the cancer, or have the antibodies made in another animal or even in a tissue culture. But by and large it doesn't work, because the genetic changes in cancer are too subtle to be detected by current immunologic techniques. With the exception of melanoma and kidney cancers, most spontaneously arising human cancers cannot be recognized by the host immune system and, therefore, immunological manipulation is not possible.

Kidney Stones

Urologists used to spend at least 10 per cent of their time dealing with stone problems. A stone blocking the urinary passage was one of life's most painful ordeals, and when there was an associated infection (a frequent occurrence), the com-bination called for immediate surgical intervention. It was one

of the few real urological emergencies. This has changed completely in recent years. Today, pulses, called shock waves, are
used to disintegrate kidney stones. Stones that will not break
up still do not mean the big 25 cm (10 inch) cut. Instead, a
pencil-size probe is inserted from the skin into the kidney core
and used to extract the stone, break it up, or provide drainage
for the urine.

The shock-wave machine has revolutionized the management of kidney stones. The shock waves are produced by a
rapidly repeating spark discharge, not unlike a sparkplug in an
automobile engine, except the discharge is in water. The
electro-hydraulic waves thus produced vaporize the fluid
between the electrodes, creating tiny, rapid shock waves that
spread out in circular fashion. As the sparks originate in an
ellipsoid container, the waves bounce off the inner wall and
create a focal point outside the ellipse, like focusing light
through a magnifying glass to burn a hole in paper. The instrument is positioned so that the stone in the kidney or ureter is
at this focal point.

Like every medical innovation, the shock-wave machine is
not a panacea for all kidney stones. As I mentioned above,
certain stones, like the pure cystine stone and certain calcium
stones, are extremely hard and do not break up well under
bombardment with shock waves. One thousand to six thousand shocks are delivered to break up each stone. Some stones
break into smaller fragments, but these fragments can be
difficult to eliminate. And even when the process has been
highly successful, stone powder can sometimes block the
drainage pipe, or there can be hypertension later on or delayed
damage to kidney function. Despite these negative notes, the
machine represents a real advance over crude surgery, which
was not free of complications either. I do not hesitate to

recommend this form of treatment to my patients. There may be a place for open operative procedure for kidney stones, but it is difficult to say when exactly.

Very large stones, estimated to be over 3 cm (approx. 1.25 inches) in diameter, are first "de-bulked." This is done by inserting a probe into the kidney like the one used to examine the inside of the bladder. Ultrasonic or laser energy is used to break up the stone, much like a pneumatic drill used to carve up pavement. The fragments are then plucked out or washed out. A catheter-size tube is left coming out of the kidney. Sand-like debris can be washed out in the subsequent days with continuous irrigation of the system. When larger fragments have been left behind, a session on the shock-wave machine or extraction of fragments with a flexible, snake-like instrument completes the job. A session on the shock-wave machine or the plucking procedure do not normally require an anaesthetic.

When the stones are smaller than 3 cm (approx. 1.25 inches) but larger than 1 cm (approx. .5 inch), a thin, hollow, wire-like tube, called a J-tube, is passed to "stent" (that is, bridge) the passage from the kidney to the bladder. A shock-wave session is followed by an X-ray two weeks later, and the J-tube is removed after all the fragments have been passed out. Stones smaller than 1 cm (approx. .5 inch) do not require a stent.

Stones in the ureter can be treated with the shock-wave machine as well. Sometimes the stone's location in the ureter makes application of shock waves difficult, as the shock waves cannot pass through bone.

Although the shock-wave machine represents a major advance in medicine, it is what might best be called end-stage technology, like the iron lung to combat polio, which was far less satisfactory than the Salk vaccine. What stone disease needs is the equivalent of a vaccine, something that can prevent stones from forming in the first place.

Investigators who have addressed this have made some progress. In about 10 per cent of cases, the actual cause of the stone formation can be determined, corrective measures instituted, and reoccurrence of the problem eliminated or rendered much less likely. But 10 per cent is not a large proportion.

Types of Stones

There are three types of kidney stones that affect the human body. (Actually, there are more than three, but the handful of others are too rare to mention here.) There are calcium-containing stones, which make up 70 per cent of all stones; struvite stones associated with bacteria that break up urea, which account for 20 per cent; and stones due to improper functioning of the body's metabolism, formed from uric acid and cystine, which account for the remaining 10 per cent.

Let us consider them in increasing order of frequency.

Cystine Stones

Cystine stones account for less than 1 per cent of all stones. They occur when the body cannot take back the amino acid cystine into the bloodstream after it has been released into the urine within the kidney.

The kidney, incidentally, works more like a pocket full of change than like an efficient filing cabinet from which the right file can be pulled out at any time. Just as you might dump out all the contents of your pants pocket before picking up the desired item, such as a dime or a subway token, the kidney dumps all the blood fluid except for the blood cells into the filtrate, and then the desired items are retrieved, one by one, and reabsorbed into the bloodstream.

When there is a cystine stone, the protein called cystine cannot be picked out and returned to the blood. This can occur as an isolated abnormality, or it can occur along with the leak of other amino acids in a condition called Fanconi syndrome. Drugs to inhibit cystine stone formation have been developed. These drugs, D-penicillamine and Theola, can be effective, but they are expensive and have side effects.

Uric Acid Stones

Uric acid stones, which represent about 10 per cent of stone disease, occur when there is excessive breakdown of nucleated cells, as when cancer, leukaemia, or lymphoma is treated. They can also occur under ordinary circumstances in people genetically predisposed to the disorder. The drug allopurinol blocks uric acid formation, and a product that precedes the formation of uric acid and is less likely to form stones becomes the final waste product. When uric acid stones have already formed, making the urine alkaline helps dissolve them, as uric acid is fourteen times more easily dissolved in an alkaline medium than in an acid or neutral urine.

Struvite Stones

When bacteria, particularly one called proteus, infects the urine, it splits the waste product urea into a chemically unstable medium that gobbles up surrounding hydrogen to stabilize itself again. When hydrogen is removed, the medium becomes highly alkaline, and in this medium struvite stones occur. Twenty per cent of all stones are of this variety. Treatment of the infection eliminates formation of new stones. For a stone that is already formed, treatment of the infection or attempts at acidification do not work; the offending stone must be eliminated first.

Calcium Stones

Seventy per cent of all kidney stones contain calcium. These stones occur when there is too much calcium in the blood, or in the urine, or both.

Sometimes it is known why blood calcium levels are too high. For example, the patient may drink an excessive amount of milk, or there may be an over-absorption of calcium from the gut, a result of excessive intake of vitamin D. For reasons less clear, a disease called sarcoidosis and beryllium poisoning are also associated with enhanced calcium absorption into the blood from the intestines.

Too much calcium can be excreted in the urine when there is increased mobilization of bone calcium, as occurs in parathyroid disease, or in any primary or secondary bone disease such as Paget's disease, bone cancer, or when the body is immobilized after an injury. Renal tubular acidosis, diabetes, hyperactive thyroid gland, and cortisone administration are other clinical conditions associated with excess calcium in the urine. But the most common cause of excess urinary calcium is "idiopathic," which means "we don't know *what* the cause is."

The distinction between excess gut uptake and excess kidney leak is made by giving a fasting patient extra calcium. This will affect the gut absorbers, not the kidney leakers. When the cause can be determined, appropriate counter-measures can be proposed. For example, patients who absorb too much calcium through their gut can be placed on a calcium-restricted diet. Patients who leak too much calcium in their kidneys can be put on hydrochlorothiazide, a drug that encourages more reabsorption of calcium into the blood-stream. Even when the cause cannot be determined, hydrochlorothiazide has proven effective in reducing the chance of further stone disease. As the drug takes calcium that might have been released in the urine back into the bloodstream, the uric acid level in the blood is increased, because it is also taken back through the same door, and thus a second drug, allopurinol, may have to be prescribed as well.

Bottom line. If you have suffered a kidney-stone attack, the chance of another attack on the same side is 20 to 25 per cent, and 10 to 15 per cent on the other side. Some people will look at these odds, conclude that a 75 per cent chance of never having another attack looks good, and elect to do nothing. Others will be alarmed at the one-in-four or one-in-five chance of another attack, and for them I recommend the following:

1. Drink enough fluids to make 2 L (3.5 pints) of urine every day. Measure the output of an average day by collecting all the urine in a bottle. Don't guess. You might be surprised how much or how little you actually pass.
2. Arrange to have a routine blood test, specifically for calcium, phosphate, parathormone, and uric acid levels.
3. Arrange an analysis of a twenty-four-hour urine collection.
4. Should there be abnormalities in either the blood or urine test, appropriate measures can be advised by your doctor.
5. If the tests are normal, you needn't make any big changes in your diet, but don't go overboard on milk and milk products such as cheese and ice cream.
6. If stones still reoccur at regular intervals, try some citrate preparations as a drink, or pills such as hydrochlorothiazide or magnesium.

Blockage

Urine flow can become blocked at any level in the urinary tract – at the kidney, at the bladder, or at the exit point. Within the kidney the blockage can be at different sites, but the problem occurs most frequently where the small sac called the renal pelvis meets the vertical pipe called the ureter. This is a uretero-pelvic junction obstruction, and leads to a swelling of the renal pelvis, a condition called hydronephrosis.

The condition can cause pain, especially when the affected kidney is forced to handle more fluid than it can cope with. The pressure build-up can damage and destroy the kidney. The condition can also be stable, when there is a swelling but with no evidence of progressive kidney damage. The degree of pain or discomfort and results of X-rays and isotope studies are used to guide the decision whether to clear the incomplete blockage.

In the most commonly performed procedure, the juncture tissue is removed, and the joint remade. Examination of the removed tissue has suggested to some experts that the problem is due to poor development of certain muscles in the area. Other investigators feel that the problem is not in the muscles but in the electrical message conducted through the system.

Like most urologists, I have carried out surgical corrections innumerable times, using different techniques and different skin incisions. Lately, I have switched over to a vertical incision in the back, an approach pioneered in Spain. This approach cuts skin, fat and ligaments but spares muscles and nerves. To me it is the most satisfactory method.

A surgical repair of a blockage that has formed scar tissue is best treated with a probe from the skin that cuts the scar using instruments like that used for stone extraction. There is a growing body of evidence to indicate that this approach may

work just as well the first time around, on a virgin uretero-
pelvic junction.

Filter Disease

There are over one million filter units, called nephrons, in
each kidney. The medical term for the filter is glomerulus, and
the disease that affects the filter is called glomerulonephritis.
It is the most common cause of kidney failure.

The disease has fascinated doctors for over a century, and,
little by little, many of its secrets have been revealed. In the
most common form of this disease, the evolution of events is as
follows: there is a bacterial throat infection with a particular
organism called streptococcus. The body reacts to this bacterial
attack with an immune response, making antibodies. These
small proteins attach to the bacterial product, the antigen, that
gave rise to them. The resulting protein-complexes, an antigen-
antibody combination, circulate throughout the bloodstream.
The complexes become trapped in the major body filter, the
glomerulus. The accumulation of the complexes creates an
injury, causing inflammation not unlike a splinter in your finger.
In 90 per cent of instances, the body overcomes the injury, the
damage to the filter is corrected, and the patient makes a full
recovery. In 10 per cent of instances, there is progressive damage
to all the filters in both organs, the kidneys fail, shrivel, and
end up as scarred, useless tissue.

We cannot as yet alter the basic course of these events, but
the search for a cure or a means of controlling the disease con-
tinues. So far, we have learned that filter disease is not caused
by all streptococcal bacteria, but by those of a particular
immunologic type. It has also been learned that an inappropriate immunologic response to white blood cells causes lupus
erythematosus, a disease that can destroy the kidney in a

fashion similar to that of the streptococcal bacteria. We have determined that the complexes deposit in different places on the filter cells. We have learned that the complexes release chemical messages that can attract certain other white blood cells or chemical agents lethal to other cells. We have tried to thwart nature's response with cortisone-type drugs, which inhibit all inflammatory responses, and tried immuno-suppressive drugs with hopes of altering body responses and anticoagulants to reduce stickiness. We have learned how to control fluid administration at different points in the disease, and to alter diet to least tax the kidney. We have devised ways to study the progress of the disease, obtaining needle-size slivers of tissue for examination under the electron microscope, obtaining magnification of one million times. It is inevitable that sooner or later we shall be able to prevent the illness, perhaps with a kind of immunization, or diminish the damaging reactions, perhaps with newer drugs, or arrest the scarring process with drugs not yet dreamed of. At least we do not have to accept the untimely and premature death of the patient as was the case before the days of dialysis and transplantation.

Dialysis

Kidneys that have shrivelled up because of the ravages of glomerulonephritis, or filter disease, cannot be distinguished from kidneys severely damaged by infection, diabetes, or high blood pressure. In this condition all kidneys look alike, and they are all useless as functional organs. But when the kidneys can't function, life can be preserved with dialysis, which substitutes for the kidneys. There are two forms of dialysis, peritoneal dialysis and haemo-dialysis.

Dialysis is a form of blood cleansing, a washing out of the unwanted accumulated waste products. In peritoneal dialysis, water is instilled into the abdomen, allowed to sit, and then drained out. Waste chemicals come out with the rinse. In haemo-dialysis, blood is pumped out of the body, into an external machine where it is washed, and then the purified blood is pumped back in. Three sessions lasting three hours each are sufficient to substitute for one week of kidney function.

Life on dialysis is never pleasant. With peritoneal dialysis there is always the threat of infection and peritonitis. Haemo-dialysis ties the patient down to the machine for seemingly endless hours. Still, life can go on.

Before the 1940s, dialysis did not exist. Patients with kidney failure were kept in a darkened room and treated with magnesium sulphate enemas in a vain effort to bring down their blood pressure. The effort seldom helped. The inevitable progression was convulsions, coma, and death.

The invention of the artificial kidney by a young Dutch doctor, Willem Kolff, has saved countless lives. It has always fascinated me that this development occurred when it did, during the Second World War, in the most war-ravaged country of all the Western nations.

Young Doctor Kolff attended a lecture on semi-permeable membranes and wondered if the principles controlling the movement of water and solids across such a membrane could not be applied to treat patients with kidney failure. He took a blood sample from a patient of his who was dying, placed it in a cellophane bag, and immersed the bag in a bath of water similar to the contents of normal body fluid. After a while, he re-analyzed the blood in the bag and found it cleansed of uraemic waste. The logical next step was to run the blood continuously through a cellophane tubing that was immersed in a bath of water, and create, in fact, an artificial kidney. Kolff's original tubing was casing obtained from a local sausage factory!

Transplantation

Kidney transplantation may be the preferred option for some patients on dialysis. If the donated kidney comes from a compatible blood relative, there is about a 90 per cent chance of maintaining satisfactory kidney function for more than 5 years. When the organ donor is unrelated, the success rate is 70 per cent, an acceptable risk, especially if a return to life on dialysis is possible in the event of transplant rejection.

The technique of kidney transplantation has not changed much from the very beginning when doctors in Boston first transplanted kidneys from one identical twin to another in the 1950s. The French surgeon Kuss first suggested placing a donated kidney into the pelvis against the pelvic bone. There was originally some concern that a kidney out of its proper position might not work as well. This was a false alarm, as was the concern that a kidney without normal nervous connections might not function adequately. The surgery consists of making three connections: the donor-kidney artery to an arterial line, often the internal iliac artery; the donor-kidney vein to a vessel in the pelvis called the iliac vein; and the donor ureter to the bladder. The vascular connections are fairly routine. Donors are usually young or middle-aged, and the vessels are pliable and workable. The ureteral connection must be done with particular care in the case of a transplant. The immuno-suppressive drugs used to prevent rejection of the graft by the body inhibit the natural healing process as well, and there can be leaks. Wound infection is also of concern. Nevertheless, transplant operations have become routine.

Matching donor to recipient and developing drug regimes, though becoming more sophisticated, have not been areas of revolutionary medical breakthrough in the last twenty-five years.

Problems inherent in kidney transplantation have not all been solved, but results have been sufficiently good to start transplanting other organs where satisfactory artificial back-up organs do not exist, such as the heart, lung, liver, or pancreas.

The first kidney transplantation in Canada took place in 1958 at the Royal Victoria Hospital, where I obtained my training and subsequently became a member of staff. I was caught up in the creative energy that pervaded the institution at the time. My hospital was among the first to launch an organ transplantation program with cadaver-source kidneys. I was still a trainee when I was sent to harvest organs from fresh cadavers. A cardiologist would nod his head to indicate that the heart had stopped, and that would signal permission for the surgeons to cut open the torso.

Christiaan Barnard and heart transplantation changed all that. Organs harvested after cardiac arrest were often damaged by lack of oxygen. This was less a problem with kidneys, because dialysis could sustain the patient until the transplant organ kicked in, but there was no such back-up for the heart. By accepting the cessation of brain waves instead of heart beats as the definition of death, doctors could harvest healthy organs for transplantation. This may have solved the legal dilemma, but, for the doctors involved, the assault on a body with a healthy heartbeat was more troublesome. The inevitable blood loss and injury to the major blood vessels would cause a brain-stem reflex resulting in a speeding of the pulse and pounding of the heartbeat. I could not help but think I was removing an organ from a body that was still protesting. Can brain waves be shocked into silence when recovery might still be possible? Was I party to legalized mayhem, if not murder? I am almost ashamed to confess we were ready to harvest kidneys from convicts after execution before Canada abolished capital punishment.

During this period, when I was well into my training in Urology, I was encouraged to help solve the problem of organ rejection. I was sent to La Jolla, California, to learn how to do a kidney transplant operation in rats. Dr. Sun Lee had developed such a model, which was being used in Dr. Frank Dixon's lab to study glomerulonephritis, or filter disease. My research director, Dr. John Dossetor, surmised that by using one inbred strain of rats as donors and another inbred strain as recipients, we would have a reproducible model that would permit the study of kidney transplantation and modification of the rejection process. Imagine my ecstacy when I solved the problem of rejection, only to find that what worked in rats could not be reproduced in another species. I did obtain a doctorate in experimental medicine, but lost much of my enthusiasm for basic research. I was ready to return, full time, to clinical practice.

Questions and Answers

- **Does swelling of the ankles mean impaired kidney function?**

The swelling can come from poor local circulation, as when the leg veins are blocked, or from a failure of the heart to pump the blood adequately, or from too much salt and water intake, as well as from kidney malfunction. When the swelling is due to kidney problems, the fluid will accumulate not only at the ankles but in the fingers and around the eyes.

- **What is creatinine, and why is the level of this substance of such concern to the nephrologist?**

Creatinine is the waste product of muscle cells. The turnover of muscle cells in the body is fairly constant. So when the level of creatinine is elevated, this is good indirect evidence of impaired kidney function. Blood urea nitrogen (BUN) levels, which reflect protein handling, serve a similar purpose, but levels of BUN can be altered by other factors, such as dehydration or blood in the gut.

- **If there is a tumour in a renal cyst, is there not a risk of spreading the cancer by needling it?**

Theoretically, that is so. In practice, kidney tumours in the needle tract hardly ever occur. Needle-tract tumours are a risk for all transitional cell carcinoma.

- **Why treat hypertension if there are no symptoms?**

When the blood pressure becomes high enough, headaches will occur and the risk of a stroke is increased.

- **The kidney cancer removed from my mother was larger than a softball, according to the doctor. She is alive and well ten years later. Was the doctor exaggerating?**

Kidney cancers can grow to the size of a softball without spread lesions. The doctor was not exaggerating, and your mother's case is not unusual.

- **I passed a kidney stone for the first time in my life at the age of forty-two. My doctor says I should be investigated only if I make another one. Is that correct?**

Most doctors would recommend a "stone work-up" only after the second stone. Nevertheless, it would not hurt to increase water intake sufficient to make 2 L (3.5 pints) of urine every day.

- **The kidney stone I had turned out to be calcium oxalate. Does that mean I should eliminate milk and milk products from my diet?**

That would make sense if you were a "milk-aholic" or if tests had shown you absorb or release excessive amounts of calcium. Otherwise, the equivalent of two glasses of milk a day should be part of a healthy diet.

- **Can an abnormal artery be the cause of an uretero-pelvic junction obstruction?**

It is not clear if an extra artery, which is common, is the cause or the effect of obstruction. When surgical correction is necessary, both issues are addressed at the time of the operation.

- **How is the choice made between dialysis and transplantation?**

When kidney function is expected to return, or if age or arterial disease rules against transplantation, dialysis is the only choice. Donor availability or personal choice may favour transplantation.

- **Are there dietary restrictions after a successful kidney transplant?**

There are no dietary restrictions if the transplanted kidney is working well. Pills to suppress rejection must be taken every day.

14

How to Take Care of Your Private Parts

Health problems, like divorces, are not matters people think out beforehand. Thus, when a problem arises, even intelligent, well-organized people become frightened and make hasty, irreversible decisions. This is especially so when the health emergency involves the groin and genital area. Reading this book has made you familiar with the workings of your genital system and kidneys and the problems that can arise. This chapter will introduce you to the health-care industry so that you can make appropriate medical decisions.

The Family Doctor

The first step is to feel comfortable with your family doctor. You have to be able to talk with him or her, if you want to. A pedantic worrier may be the right doctor for one individual, and a confident, parental type more appropriate for another. You may not feel comfortable with a doctor who acts as a first-aid station and sends every patient to a specialist. On the other hand, you may feel that your doctor assumes too much responsibility and doesn't refer patients to appropriate specialists soon enough. You may want to talk things out in detail with your doctor, or you may prefer to know only what is necessary. But whatever your choice, your doctor mustn't intimidate you. You should feel that you can be at ease talking to him or her about what are normally private matters. Since you cannot change the practice style of a doctor, the wisest thing to do if there is a problem is to change doctors.

Once you have found your doctor, make sure he or she is focused on your health problem. A doctor should be interested in your occupation, but if you say that you are an auto mechanic, and he or she has been having a problem with an alternator, you shouldn't spend all the time talking about car problems and neglect the real purpose of your visit. There is nothing wrong in making a friend of your doctor, but keep your medical problem in focus.

And be leery of psychological dismissals. It is widely recognized that as many as 90 per cent of all visits to family doctors are for stress or emotional problems. Unless the disease is clear-cut, there is a natural tendency for primary physicians to label problems as psychological. Impotence, for example, is easily dismissed as being stress- or age-related. But if you are prematurely and unjustifiably saddled with the judgement that your trouble is psychosomatic, tell the doctor that you don't want your epitaph to read: "I told you bastards I was sick."

How to Be a Good Patient

Sometimes people take extraordinary steps to deny a problem that may already be present. I remember a patient who first came to see me because he saw blood in his urine. Tests showed a bladder tumour, which was removed. But the patient knew that bladder tumours are often a recurrent problem and that blood in the urine can be an early sign of the disease. After the operation he began urinating in total darkness so that he could not see the colour of his urine. At the other extreme are patients who imagine every sickness, such as the patient who drinks too much tea, urinates twice in the night, and thinks he has a prostate problem. These extremes are counterproductive. To get the best care possible, what is needed is an informed, levelheaded approach.

Your Medical History

The patient is, potentially, a resource in his or her own health care, and prepared patients can help the doctor zero in on the right diagnosis and treatment. Beware the doctor who is not interested in your past illnesses, because he is ignoring the fundamentals of history-taking, as taught in medical school. A thorough doctor takes detailed notes on your body history, which tells him or her if a health problem is a reoccurrence of an old ailment, something related to the old problem, or something new and unrelated. A doctor should also consider your family history, because certain illnesses tend to occur more often in certain families, which is not surprising since families share genes and experiences.

Keep a list of all past illnesses that required hospitalization – when they occurred, what the diagnosis was, what treatment was followed, and what the outcome was. If you are taking medication for hypertension, it may be causing your impotence. Decongestants may prevent you from urinating. Any manipulation of the urethra may be the cause of infection. A family history of diabetes, cancer, or heart disease is significant, as is a history of unsolved family illness. I have seen more undescended testicles in siblings than in the general population, and hernias occur more often in some families than in others. A doctor can't help responding to a challenge, so, by all means, stimulate his or her intellectual curiosity.

Medications and Allergies

Make a list of the drugs, with their dosages, that you are taking. Don't rely on your ability to describe them, or your memory. I remember this unfortunate exchange:

"What medications are you taking?"

"I take a pink pill in the morning, then a blue pill and a white pill every second day."

"Do you know the names of these pills?"

"No, I remember them by the colour."

"Can we call your drugstore?"

"I forget which one I went to. It's on the bottle, but I don't have the bottle with me."

Can you imagine the service such a patient is likely to receive compared to the patient who appears with a carefully prepared list of medications? Unless your doctor knows what you are taking, you cannot begin a new treatment. He or she cannot risk a drug combination that may be harmful.

A list of allergies is also useful, especially in the case of people who have already had a dangerous drug reaction or are prone to allergies. Asthmatic people, people with hay fever, and people who are allergic to household articles or pets are more likely than others to have allergic reactions to chemicals injected for diagnostic tests, such as dyes used to show up the heart vessels or to outline the urinary tract.

The Surgeon

If you have consulted with your family doctor, explored alternatives, and have then decided to have prostate or other surgery, the choice of a surgeon is your next important decision. It is wise to remember that, even when you are sick, you have options. Just because there is only one urological surgeon in town, for example, does not mean that you are obliged to stay in that town. And even if your family doctor has gone to the trouble of making arrangements for surgery to be undertaken by a particular surgeon in a particular hospital, whom he or she describes as "the very best," you are not bound by that arrangement. You may not feel confident or comfortable with your doctor's choice, or the surgeon may have operated unsuccessfully on someone close to you and you therefore have misgivings. My feeling is that even if they are superstitions, you may be wise to respond to your misgivings. Exercising these options may seem impolite, but having records transferred to another hospital, or another doctor, are a patient's privilege.

Schooling

You may wonder whether it is important to find out what school your surgeon attended, or how he or she stood in his class? Certainly it is true that medical schools such as Harvard or Johns Hopkins have enormous reputations, unquestionably well-deserved. But a school or institution earns its reputation through the quality and quantity of its research, not through its teaching of medical students. And a teacher in a medical school is hardly ever appointed because of an ability to teach. He or she is assigned the task on the basis of research published, and because somebody has to do it.

An extraordinarily bright student might do best in a name school, as he or she will be exposed to the latest and newest developments in the different disciplines. An average student, on the other hand, will get little help weeding out the pertinent material. On the whole, smaller schools do the basic, didactic teaching better. My conclusion after seeing a generation of medical students and hospital residents is that the individual factor far outweighs the institutional factor. Often, a

superior student from a little school becomes a better specialist than a mediocre student from a large and famous school.
Furthermore, performance as a medical student does not indicate how one will perform as a specialist. Skills, such as the
hand-eye co-ordination necessary in carving out the prostate
or the three-dimensional perception essential in difficult
cancer surgery, cannot possibly be assessed in an undergradu-
ate medical-school program. Bedside manners can be learned,
but real warmth and sensitivity cannot.

As a patient I would not worry what school my surgeon
attended, nor how he or she performed as a student, although
a surgeon must have the basic credentials.

Credentials

Since each country qualifies its surgeons in its own way, pres-
tigious-sounding degrees and titles have to be put in context.

In England, Scotland, and Ireland, surgeons-in-training
take their qualifying exams early in the training program.
Those who pass can add F.R.C.S. (Fellow of the Royal College
of Surgeons) to their name. If the exam was taken in
Edinburgh, the letters are followed by a bracketed E, if in
Ireland, by a bracketed I, and so on. Because a doctor in Britain
can take the Fellowship exam before completing his or her
training, a British Fellowship does not necessarily mean a
doctor is a fully trained surgeon. The Fellowship only means
that the doctor has passed the exam that allows him or her to
compete for Registrars, a scarce resident's position in a teaching hospital. After several years, a Registrar becomes a senior
Registrar and is, finally, a fully trained surgeon. At this point a
surgeon can assume a Consultant position, but these are few
and far between and become available, for the most part, only
when someone retires or dies.

In Canada, would-be surgeons must first graduate from

medical school. They then take a minimum of five years of approved surgical training, and, after the training is complete, they must successfully pass a gruelling set of Fellowship examinations. The Fellowship finals consist of three sessions, two relating to clinical practice and one relating to the basic sciences. A failure rate of 25 to 50 per cent is not unusual. One of my old professors once said that the guys who struggled to pass become "the bastards" when they are the examiners. Those who pass the Fellowships may add F.R.C.S.C. to their name. Those who don't pass can try again two more times. If they fail three times, they usually revert to general practice or must take further training before they can sit the exams again.

In the United States, surgeons become qualified by sitting for state exams during and after five years of approved training. Those who pass become Board Certified surgeons; those who don't can still pass themselves off as specialists, being "board eligible." Once a Board Certified surgeon has practised long enough to have a track record of major cases, he or she may apply for Fellowship, an honorary title. The surgeon presents documentation of his or her cases and takes an oral exam, but at this point becoming an American Fellow (F.A.C.S.) is rather routine.

Basically, in Britain, Canada, and the United States, a surgeon is a doctor who has graduated from medical school and has taken a minimum of five years' additional training. Not too long ago, there was considerable reciprocity between countries. British senior Registrars, Canadian Fellows, and American Board Certified surgeons could apply for equivalent status in any of the three countries. Recently, rules about licensing have become more rigid, and each country expects new immigrants to take extra years of training.

Reputation

The reputation of a surgeon within a hospital or a community does not necessarily mean exceptional skills or competence. It may reflect personal charm, affability, availability – even fee structure. The government medicare program in Canada has made variable fees obsolete, but before that my fee schedule was moderate, and for this reason I *lost* a number of patients. They thought that doctors who charged three times as much must be three times as good. Fees in many countries are arbitrarily set, not governed by any professional or government regulations, and certainly do not reflect services, promised or rendered.

The Choice

Neither schooling, credentials, nor word-of-mouth reputation means as much as how the surgeon performs daily. I have come to the conclusion that perhaps the best way to choose a surgeon is to ask the hospital staff – nurses, anaesthetists, doctors – whom they consider a good surgeon. Whom would they choose if they required a particular operation or care? They have seen the doctor in action and under stress and they know the results. There is no doubt that the hospital staff is the best judge of a surgeon's skill.

Community versus University Hospital

If you are scheduled for major surgery at a community hospital, would you be better off at a large university centre? The primary consideration should be medical expertise and the question of a transfer should, certainly, be considered. If the suggestion is welcomed but valid reasons offered why it is not necessary, you might be persuaded to stay. The community hospital might, for example, point out that they have performed your particular procedure hundreds of times and that their complication rate is only 6 per cent compared to the reported 12 per cent average. In general, this kind of information is reassuring, although I must confess that I have heard doctors lie about figures. I was shocked at a court hearing once, when a surgeon who was called as an expert witness for the defence to testify about a vesico-vaginal fistula (a hole between the vagina and bladder), said that he had looked after cases such as this "hundreds of times." I knew that in a ten-year period there had been dozens, not hundreds, of such cases in major American centres. When I objected, the doctor reminded me that "we have to protect our colleagues from unnecessary litigations." The incident gives pause for thought.

If the community hospital convinces you that it has the requisite medical expertise, you may elect to stay. And familiar surroundings, friendly staff, proximity to home, better parking facilities, and better visiting hours are also reasons (albeit less compelling) for choosing a particular hospital.

There is an old saying that "those who can, do; and those who can't, teach." Reasoning this way, some patients think that university teaching hospitals have mediocre surgeons. It could be that a busy, unaffiliated surgeon might, possibly, hone his skills more than a university professor who also teaches, supervises research, and does administrative work. But there are two major reasons why I would choose a university hospital for major surgery. First, the justification for any procedure is more strictly controlled. In a community hospital, operations of questionable merit can go unchallenged; in a teaching hospital, surgical decisions are subject to the scrutiny of medical students, resident doctors, and the surgeon's peers. A hasty or incorrect diagnosis based on poor or inadequate justifications will become a topic of debate in a teaching hospital, if not of ridicule. Second, I would feel safer in a hospital where resident doctors are in attendance at all hours. When author-surgeon William A. Nolen needed coronary by-pass surgery, he chose a university teaching hospital, not, he says, because he thought the surgeon was superior, but because the resident doctors were there around the clock. It made sense to him and it makes sense to me.

There is one other troublesome issue I must discuss. Many well-meaning people suggest you should choose a surgeon with extensive experience in a particular surgical procedure, like radical prostatectomy. A renowned religious leader who had undergone the procedure makes this suggestion in an essay he was asked to prepare after his ordeal. His son-in-law, a Urology resident at the time, showed me the essay. "What your father-in-law is saying," I said, "is that I must hoard all the cases and not allow the residents to get any training." Dr. Patrick Walsh, who devised a nerve-sparing method of radical prostatectomy, makes the same recommendation in his new book. But how are we going to train the coming generation of surgeons if all the staff in the teaching hospitals assume that stance? Aren't we saying to patients: "Let someone else be the guinea pig"?

I think surgery at the teaching hospitals should be done by senior residents under staff supervision. Certainly there may be instances when the staff should have intervened earlier, but by and large there is little difference in the outcome, no matter who actually held the scalpel. Surgery is a team effort, and too much blame or credit should not be attributed to any one individual.

The Patient-Doctor Interaction

There are patients who always complain about their previous doctor, and I suspect they complain about me when they move on to the next. There are patients who are never critical of any doctors, and patients who are forever fearful. There are glum patients, and there are cheerful patients, a doctor's delight. Doctors are human and are likely to be nice to people who are nice to them. Doctors are also professionals and appreciate it when a patient is helpful in diagnosis and co-operative in treatment.

I must confess that I get annoyed when patients cannot give me a straight answer to a simple question:

"How many times do you have to empty your bladder during the night?"

"Well, that depends, Doctor."

"Depends on what?"

"How much I have drunk."

"Say, on an average day."

"I have no average day."

"How many times did you get up to go to the bathroom last night?"

"Last night?"

"Yes, last night."

"Well, you'll have to ask my wife that."

"Why?"

"She's more likely to notice that kind of thing."

"Did you get up at all?"

"Oh, yes."

"But you can't tell me how often?"

"Let me see, what day was it yesterday?"

"Yesterday was Monday."

"I think it was Sunday when we had a visit from my brother

and his wife. I had some coffee, which I never should have done, and I was up all night. Of course, it was all my fault. I didn't have to, I could have declined. But it didn't seem polite not to. Everybody else was having coffee. . . . What was that you were asking?"

If one simple question leads to this type of exasperating exchange, the doctor will be totally frustrated by the time he has the full and accurate story, upon which he must base 90 per cent of his diagnosis.

It is also frustrating when patients do not follow a course of treatment. Consider this exchange:

"I'm not better, Doctor."

"I'm sorry. I was so certain the pills I prescribed would help you."

"Well, I must tell you I didn't take all those pills."

"You didn't?"

"The last time a doctor gave me pills to take, I got so sick. I was afraid it might happen again. I took half a pill for a few days. It didn't make me better, so I stopped."

"I'm sorry I didn't impress upon you how important it was to take the pills in the dosage prescribed."

"I'm sure you did, Doctor, but I was frightened. Can we try it again?"

The Second Opinion

After surgery has been suggested, should you seek a second opinion?

In my estimation, you should raise the question of a second opinion, if only to test the reaction. If your doctor becomes difficult, abusive, aggressive, uneasy, or seems to feel threatened, you should certainly insist upon a second opinion. On the other hand, if your doctor welcomes the suggestion and helps you in every possible way, I might wonder if it is actually necessary. Most surgeons with whom I work, when faced with a controversial or complicated problem, raise the possibility of a second opinion before it is suggested by the patient. When the question is not raised, it is usually because there is little to be gained by it. Still, if for some reason you lose faith or confidence in your surgeon, make the change. After all, it is your life and your health we are talking about.

People rarely think of taking preventive measures for their own health, although they are careful to arrange immunization for their children against polio, diphtheria, whooping cough, tetanus, measles, and the like. Yet there are measures you can take to safeguard your health.

Hospitals and health care are often governed by secret unwritten laws. The universal medicare program in Canada, for example, means that doctors are paid for what they do, not for how well they do it. This means that a doctor who does three good circumcisions and two sloppy ones will collect the same fee as a doctor who does five perfect circumcisions. The medicare system can only count, it does not measure quality. Therefore, make sure you really need the suggested procedure and that you have picked the doctor to do it properly. In the United States, private insurance often means that the doctor gets higher fees when more tests are done. Your strategy in getting good care should take note of that. You can ask your doctor why he or she has ordered each test and what information each will provide. If your doctor has to justify the tests, he or she will be prudent. You might also want to explore reasons for a referral. Is it a referral to a golf buddy, or is it based on past results? And it is often wise not to ask for special considerations. When the normal hospital routine is upset, more things can go wrong. I suspect that is why there are more complications when relatives of doctors are the patients.

P.S.

Look after your health. Your overall physical condition will affect the health of your private parts. Don't throw away the well-being you have been given. Rather, take care of yourself with good diet and regular exercise. In general, people smoke too much, drink too much, sit too much, and eat too much, when they know all too well that these habits are detrimental to their health. Smoking, for example, causes not only lung cancer but also bladder cancer. It also constricts all the small blood vessels of the body and can, by constricting the small artery to the penis, cause impotence. It is good practice, especially for the health of the prostate gland, to eat less, particularly less red meat, and instead to consume fish, white poultry meat, fibre, vegetables, and fruit. It is healthy to exercise more and worry less. Keep tabs on your health and clear records of any medical events. If you take care of yourself and are a resourceful, aware patient you are doing the best you can. The medical profession provides a specific scientific resource, but ultimately you must be responsible for your own health.

Index

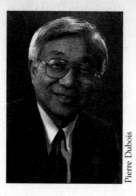

Pierre Dubois

DR. YOSH TAGUCHI is Program Director of Urology at McGill University and a senior urologist at Royal Victoria Hospital in Montreal. In addition to publishing in scientific journals (*Journal of Urology, Urology, British Journal of Urology, CMAJ*, and *Canadian Journal of Surgery*), he has contributed articles in *Geriatrics, Diagnosis*, and *The Canadian Doctor*.

MERRILY WEISBORD is a writer and broadcaster living in Montreal. She is the author of *The Strangest Dream: Canadian Communists, the Spy Trials and the Cold War* (1983, 2nd ed. 1994) and *Our Future Selves: Love, Life, Sex, and Aging* (1991), and is co-author of *The Valour and the Horror: The Untold Story of Canadians in the Second World War* (1991).

If you would like further specific information about a urological problem, starting in September 1996 you can reach Dr. Taguchi through the Internet and the World Wide Web at the following address:

http://www.mediconsult.com

There is a fee for this service and it is not covered under any government health plan.